Work Your Wardrobe

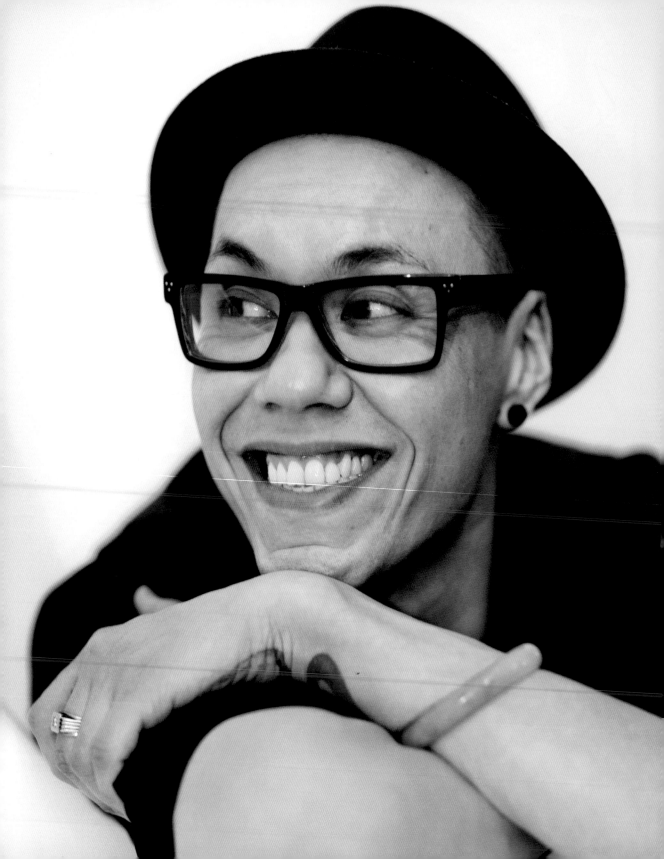

GOK WAN

Work Your Wardrobe

Gok's Gorgeous Guide to Style That Lasts

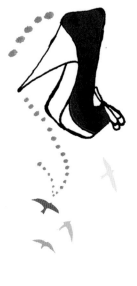

HarperCollins*Publishers*

HarperCollins*Publishers*
77–85 Fulham Palace Road,
Hammersmith, London W6 8JB
www.harpercollins.co.uk

First published by HarperCollins*Publishers* 2009
This edition 2010

10 9 8 7 6 5 4 3 2 1

© Gok Wan 2009

Edited by Caragh McKay

Photography:
© Perou 2009

Reportage Photography:
© Chris Gloag 2009

Additional Portrait Photography:
© Adam Lawrence 2009

Still Life Photography:
© Benoît Audureau 2009
© Objective Image 2009

Illustration:
© Kat Heyes 2009

Art Directed and Designed by Nikki Dupin

ISBN: 978-0-00-731853-7

Printed and bound in China by South China Printing Co. Ltd.

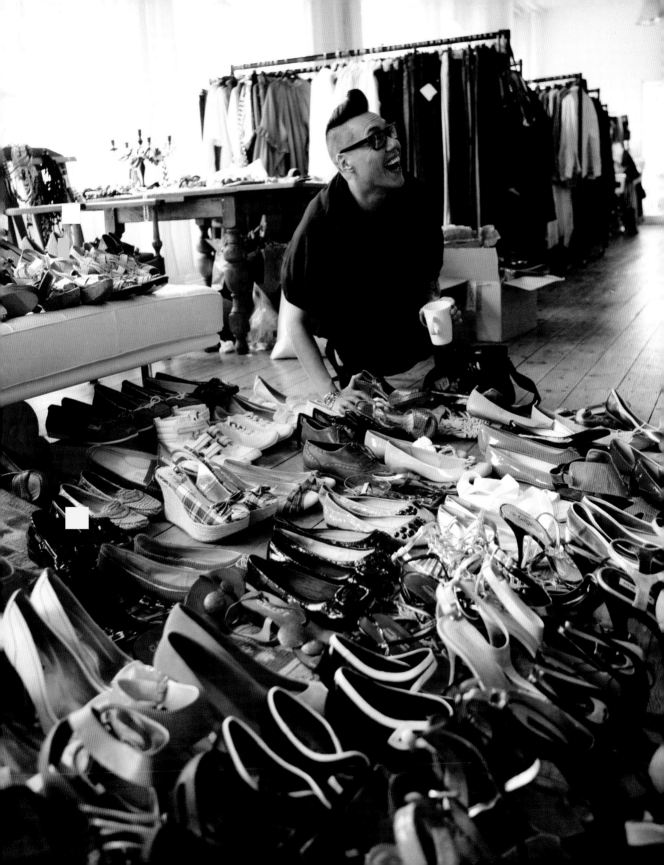

contents

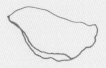

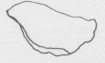

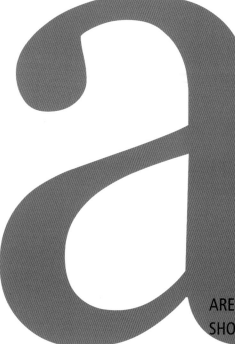

ARE YOU ONE OF MY GIRLS WHO GOES OUT SHOPPING EVERY SATURDAY, HAS A WARDROBE PACKED FULL OF CLOTHES BUT NOTHING TO WEAR? THEN READ ON, MY DARLING, BECAUSE ALL THAT'S ABOUT TO CHANGE. We are going to take a fresh look at what you wear, and I am going to show you how to put together some great new outfits that you will love. What's more, my stylish sweethearts, you won't have to spend, spend, spend to do it!

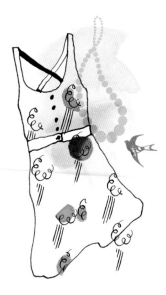

8

British women shell out an average of £1,000 a year on clothes!

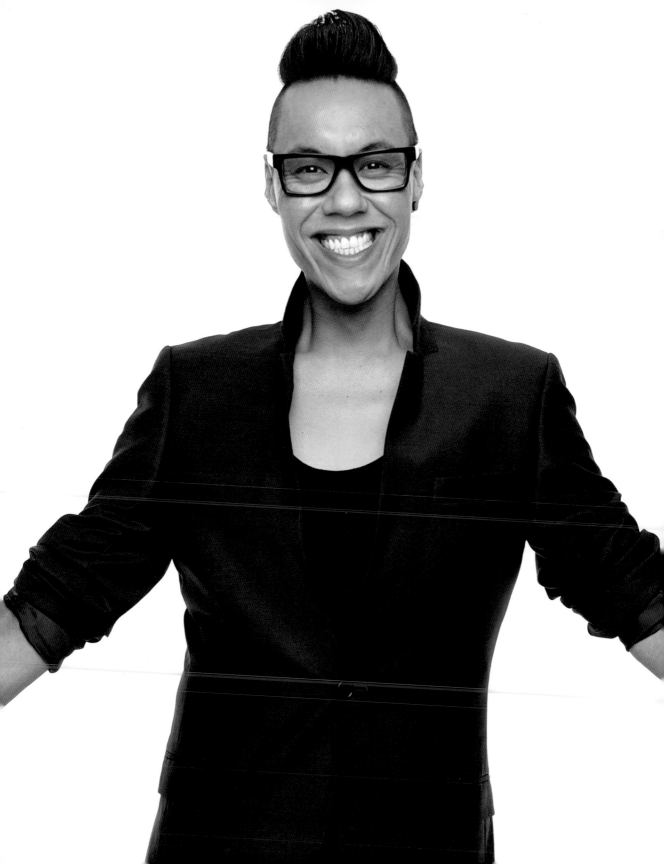

British women shell out an average £1,000 a year on clothes and yet only a third of those fashion finds ever sees the light of day. The rest, it seems, are banished to the dark recesses of your wardrobes, along with all those other pieces that fashion forgot. Nearly every girl's wardrobe that I see (and let's face it, my angels, I have seen more than most!) is bursting with clothes that have never been worn. And that's where my style quest to get you to buy less and wear more comes in.

So, girl, walk over to that wardrobe right now, throw open the doors and, like discovering your own little Narnia, get ready to step into the magical world within. Here's where we start sorting out the good from the bad and the ugly, decide what to keep, what to add, and – most important of all, girls – what to kiss goodbye to. (I know how hard it is, gorgeous, but believe me, it really is for the best!)

"Nearly every girl's wardrobe that I see is bursting with clothes that have never even been worn."

Whether it's those trusty black trousers, that one-for-all winter coat or those sparkly slingbacks that you paid a fortune for but have never worn, I am going to be right by your side revisiting everything you have got stuffed away in there.

We'll do all this while keeping an eye on the latest trends, of course, and I'll give you loads of advice on how to create a classic collection of outfits along the way. I also want all the tips and tricks in this book to inspire you beautiful belles to break free of any dressing habits that are way past their sell-by date, and to try out something new, because a change of direction will always spruce up your style.

Just remember, ladies, when it comes to being truly stylish, there really are no hard and fast rules: you can pick and choose elements of any outfit and adapt them to suit your look. Whether you are a trend-savvy teenager, a thirtysomething career girl or a fabulous fiftysomething, this book is all about building a brilliantly hard-working wardrobe, and that means a wardrobe that works for you.

I'll show you how to create the kind of simple style statements that never go out of fashion, that you can adapt to suit your size and shape, and that you can depend on to make you feel your beautiful best every day. I'm not suggesting that shopping sprees are off the agenda, though, girls – we all want to feel part of what's going on in fashion – I just want you to see how easy it is to look and feel fabulous without breaking the bank.

To help you get the most out of our new style journey, and so that you can quickly revisit the parts that work best for you, I've split this book into four easy-to-find sections. In SECTION 1, we'll put some solid fashion foundations in place as I

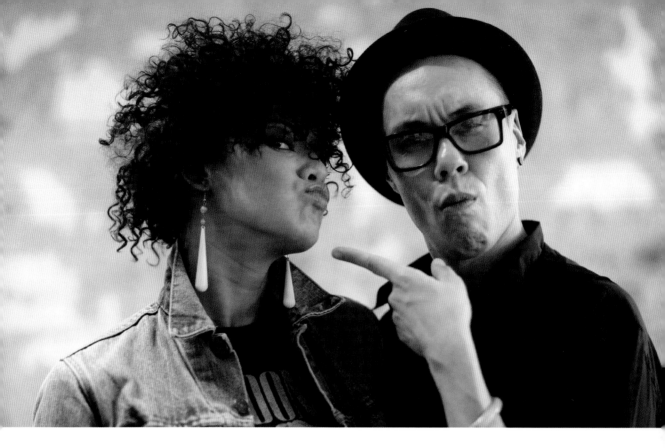

highlight the key pieces of clothing that I think no woman should be without. SECTION 2 is where we compile the ultimate accessories drawer and discover why the devil really is in the detail. In SECTION 3, I'll use my stylist know-how to show you how to create a timeless selection of gorgeously chic outfits, and in SECTION 4, we'll add a slick of gloss and polish to your fab new outfits with some gorgeous hair and make-up tips.

And that's it. By making your wardrobe work for you, you'll be a collection of chic new looks richer and ready to feel fashion fabulous anytime, anyplace, anywhere. Because the one thing you never, ever have to cut back on is feeling gorgeous. That, my angels, doesn't cost a thing.

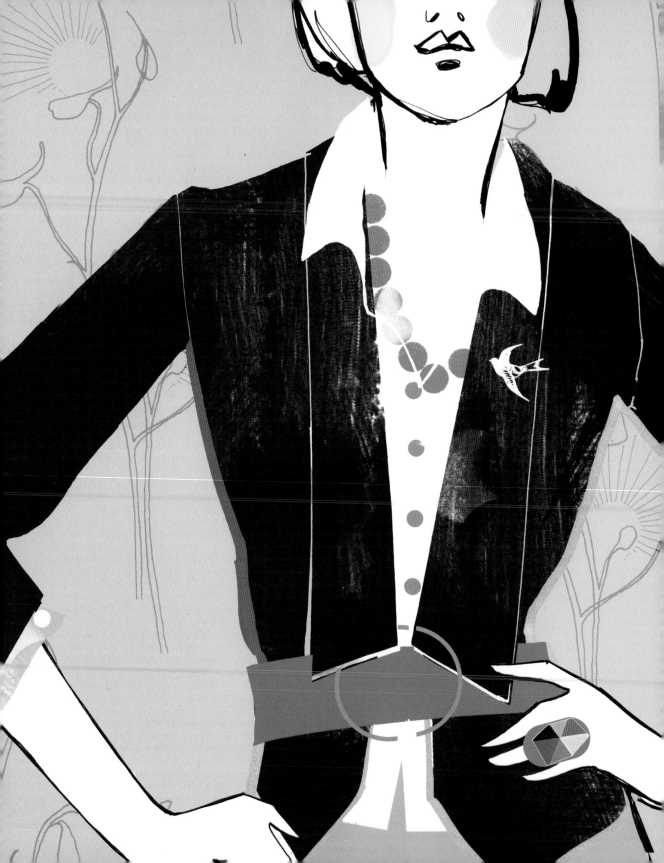

chic classics

From white shirts to pencil skirts and
the classic mac, in this section we've got
the basics covered

the white shirt

THERE'S A LOT MORE TO THIS SIMPLE *piece of wardrobe kit than you might think, girls. And, no matter how you like to wear your white shirt, trust me, by the time you've finished this chapter, you'll be pulling it out of your wardrobe and wearing it a whole lot more.*

The white shirt has got such fabulous fashion potential!

THE WHITE SHIRT IS A TRUE CLASSIC. THE MINUTE YOU FIND ONE THAT YOU LIKE it becomes your new best friend – you can always depend on it. But like anything we come to know and love, ladies, sometimes we can take the white shirt a teensy bit for granted. All you smart girls will undoubtedly have a white shirt in your wardrobe, but I'll bet if I asked you how you wore it, you would probably say that it was mostly for work. Yet it's got such fabulous style potential. Think of **Marilyn Monroe** in *The Misfits* wearing a man's white shirt with simple jeans – she looks red hot! And that's how your white shirt should make you feel.

Let's take a look at **THREE CLASSIC WHITE-SHIRT STYLES**, and over the next couple of pages I'll share my top tips on how to wear them.

1 *the classic*

THE MOST TRADITIONAL SHIRT SHAPE OF ALL IS CLEAN, CRISP AND SMART, AND WILL ALWAYS SAY 'ELEGANT CITY CHIC'. The minute you pair it with a suit jacket and trousers, though, it can look a little too traffic-warden chick. (Come on – even all you lovely wardens out there will admit that this is not a look you'd go for if you had the choice!) So let's clock in and whip that 'work-uniform' element right out of the classic white by loosening it up and bringing it bang up to date.

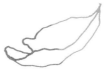

• NATURAL BEAUTY

Dressing down is the new dressing up and this look nails that style perfectly. Opt for a shirt that's a size or two bigger and you've got classic boyfriend style. Or just nick one from your other half and give it a soft, feminine touch. (Don't worry, he won't notice – until he sees how fab you look in it! Girls look so sexy in oversized men's shirts.) Because this is the perfect look for casual days, just wear it as big and baggy as you want, then raid your accessories drawer and add a few girlie touches – quilted ballet pumps and some long necklaces, say. If you are going to be heading out for drinks at some point, style it plain and loose over smart ankle-skimming trousers with some high, high heels. Or just pair it with your favourite denims and boots for a *très* sexy look.

• UPTOWN GIRL

This is all about classic workwear with a sharp, sexy edge, and it's a style that I think looks good on women of any shape and age. The shirt should skim your figure, not cling to it. And let's give those suit trousers that you pull out for work every day a rest for a while. Pull out a figure-enhancing

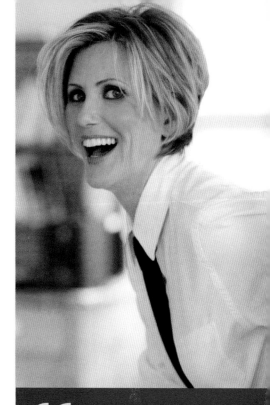

> **66**
> *Dressing down is the new dressing up and this look nails that style perfectly.*
> **99**

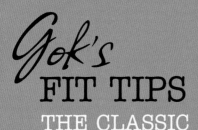

Gok's FIT TIPS

THE CLASSIC

1. GORGEOUS PEARS
A classic white shirt will show off your ladylike waist, and if your shirt has a wide collar, it will balance out your bottom half.

2. CURVY CHICKS
Keep it baggy around the waist and buttoned low at the neckline, as this will slim down your top half, reduce the cling factor around your tummy and focus all attention on your Betty Grable-like pins!

3. PETITE PRINCESS
Be careful not to go too big or baggy, as that will just swamp your dainty frame, and, let's face it, the tent was never a good look, especially on you, gorgeous!

> " My beautiful darlings, don't forget to pull up your sleeves. You'll be amazed at how it changes your look! "

pencil skirt instead. (I'm sure you've got one hanging in there, sassy girl.) Wear your shirt with a fitted waistcoat (**Victoria Beckham** pulls this look off beautifully), roll up the sleeves and add heels and a slim patent belt (or any of your trusted big, sexy waist-cinchers) to show you mean business.

20

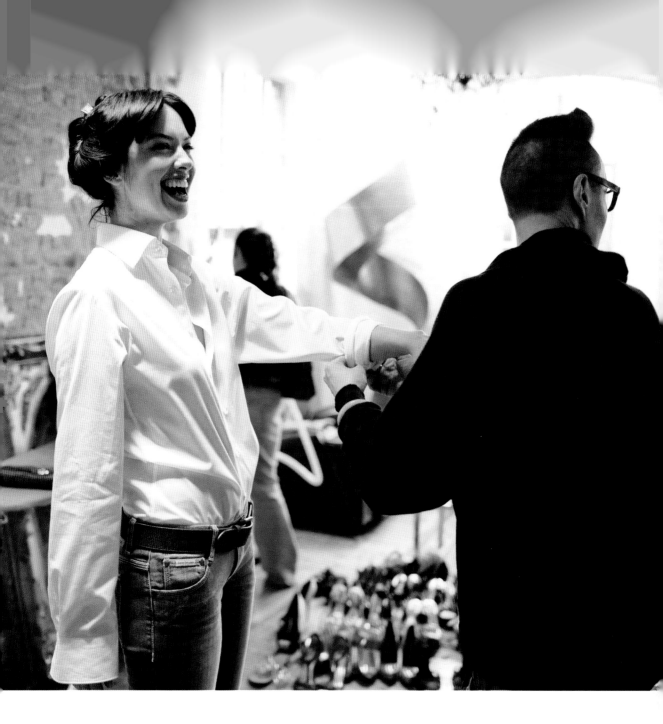

21

THE WHITE SHIRT

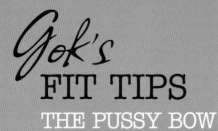

Gok's FIT TIPS
THE PUSSY BOW

1. This extra-ladylike look is a great one for my sexy girls who are slim on top: there's so much detail going on around the top half that your elegant neck will be the focus point.

2. If you don't like the idea of being too buttoned up, or looking like a nun in *The Sound of Music*, undo the top button, leave the neck open and let the ties hang soft and loose around the neckline.

3. Different fabrics create different styles: silky pussy bow blouses have a sophisticated feel, while cotton versions will be crisp and cool for the office or look fab dressed down with jeans.

2 *the pussy bow*

A BIG, BEAUTIFUL, FLOPPY BOW AT THE NECKLINE OF YOUR SHIRT ADDS A WHOLE NEW DIMENSION TO CLASSIC OFFICE STYLE – not to mention a much needed flash of glamour around the photocopier. It's also a great office-to-bar option. If your pussy bow has detachable ties, all the better: you're getting two blouses for one. One shirt, so many options – gorgeous!

• NICE AND SIMPLE

Loosen the bow so that the ties hang down in a knot just above your bust, tuck the shirt into that pair of favourite straight-cut blue jeans and wear a cardie casually on top. Popping out to lunch with the girls? Slip on those do-all ballet pumps and pull the look together with any of your handbags that have buckles or metal detail on them – in black, brown or tan – for a *soupçon* of French chic.

22

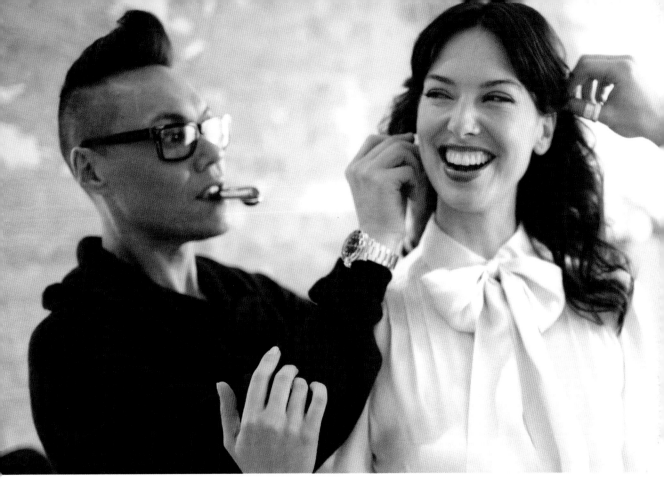

• GORGEOUSLY GIRLIE

You can really go over the top on the prettiness of this style by tying the bow as big and flouncy as possible at the neck – think of it as a gorgeous big ribbon – and pairing it with a girlie shaped skirt. A tulip or a bell style skirt would look the business, too. Don't forget to add that all-important va va voom factor with a pair of your favourite stilettos. High-waisted trousers would also look good if you prefer not to wear skirts. Silky pyjama-style pants will ooze Old Hollywood glamour – think Katharine Hepburn – paired with some great wedge heels.

1. The wrapover shirt will suit all my busty beauties who would prefer not to look too top-heavy: it will flatter your gorgeous curves in all the right places. A three-quarter-length sleeve version will balance your shape by focusing attention on your small waist.

2. The plunging V-neck of a wrapover makes it a perfect option for any of you ladies who say 'no' to diets but who want to make your top half look slimmer, as it has a narrowing effect.

3. If you are one of my girls who has that annoying problem of shirts gaping across the bust, the wrap is for you.

3 *the wrap*

I KNOW THAT LOADS OF MY GIRLS LIKE THIS STYLE FOR WORK, AND I THINK THAT THE WRAP IS A GREAT ALTERNATIVE TO THE CLASSIC WHITE SHIRT. It always looks smart and city-like, but doesn't feel too buttoned up, so it's the perfect style for all you ladies who like a more relaxed look.

• A CHOICE CLASSIC

This is a great style for the office or for off-duty days. To stop it looking too matronly (some wrap shirts can have an ageing effect by making you look too square on top, so watch out!), go for a wrap with detail, such as an extra-wide collar or big, puffy sleeves. Pair it with black three-quarter-length narrow – or cigarette – pants and plain pumps for Audrey Hepburn-esque chic.

The wrap is a great alternative to the classic white shirt . . . it's a great option for all my older girls who like a more relaxed look.

• NIGHT AND THE CITY

A wrap shirt tucked into a sexy pencil skirt and – at the point where the shirt crosses over – pinned with a big, glam brooch looks fab for evening. Accessorising like this has been a real trend on the catwalks lately – it reminds me of those sexy Givenchy styles. The most brilliant thing about this outfit, though, is that it's so easy to pull off: just pin a brooch on to your shirt, leave your jacket hanging loosely over your shoulders, sling on a pair of black stilettos and, beautiful, you're ready to sashay on into cocktail hour.

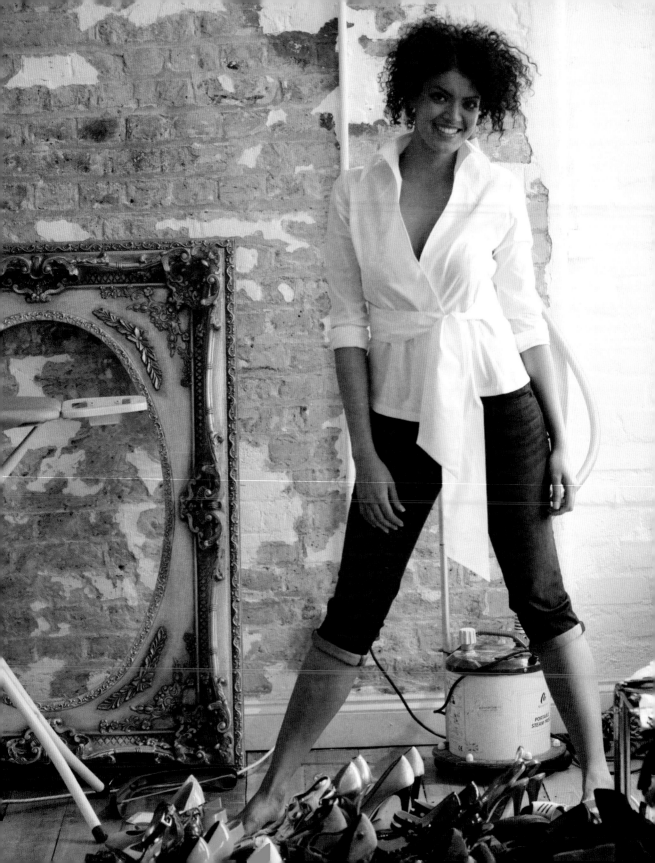

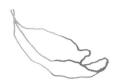

" The wrap will flatter your curves in all of the right places. It also has a narrowing effect at the waist. Gorgeous! "

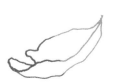

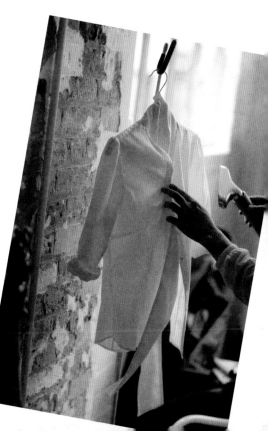

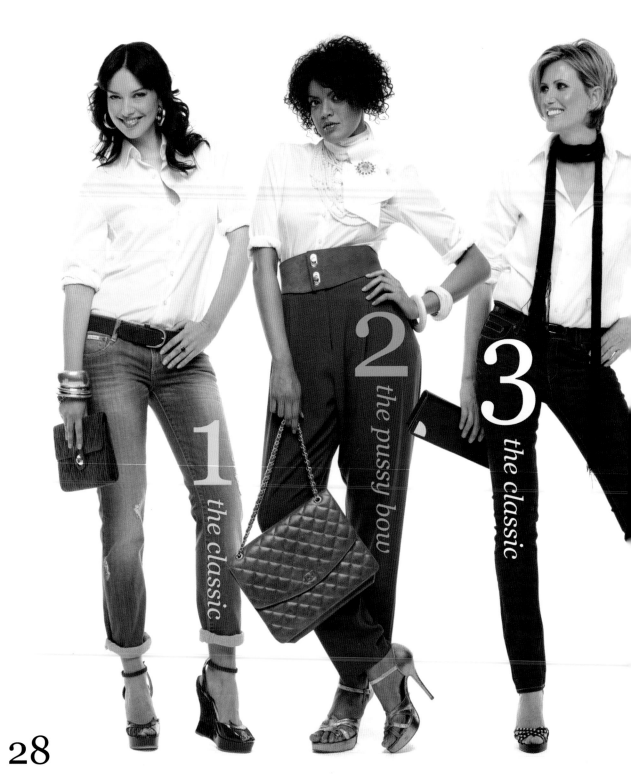

1 the classic

2 the pussy bow

3 the classic

28

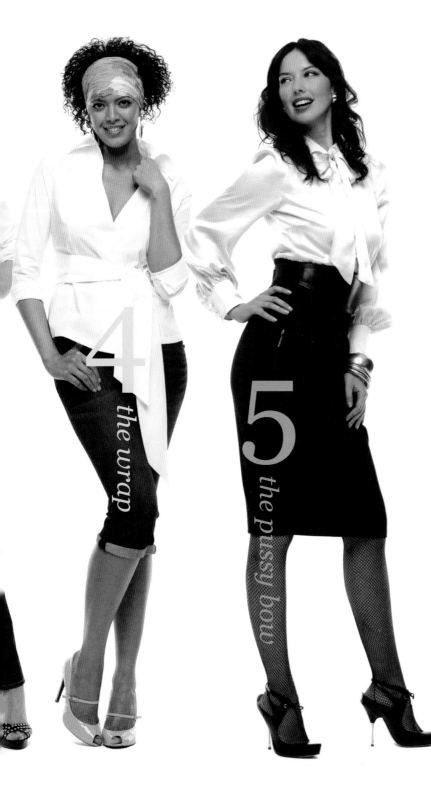

4 *the wrap*

5 *the pussy bow*

> The white shirt is a true classic. Like your best friend, you can always depend on it.

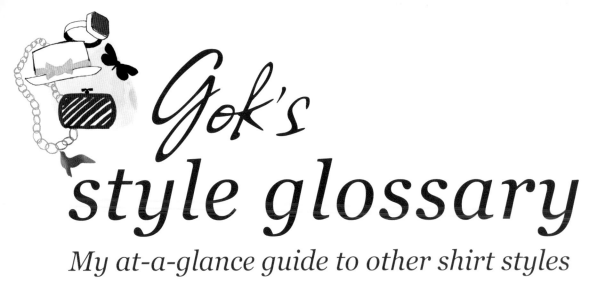

Gok's style glossary

My at-a-glance guide to other shirt styles

THE GRANDAD

- **THE LOOK:** this straight-up-and-down collarless style says casual cool – perfect for girls who don't like the stiffness of a fitted white shirt.

- **WEAR WITH:** jeans and some plain thong sandals, plus a pair of big hoop earrings – so simple. So sexy!

- **GOOD FIT FOR:** curvy girls who want to cover the tummy area – try one with a little smocking to stop it clinging. Petites should get as neat a fit as possible so that your shirt draws attention to your shape in all the right ways.

- **NOT THE BEST FIT FOR:** juicy pears – if your shirt's too narrow at the top, it will set your shape off balance.

- **FAMOUS FOR WORKING THE LOOK:** preppy A-listers, such as Gywneth Paltrow and Jennifer Aniston.

> **"**
> *Wear with a big pair of hoop earrings. So simple. So sexy!*
> **"**

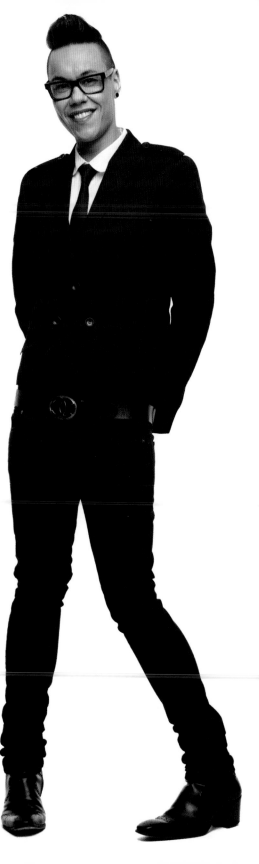

No matter how you wear it, your white shirt should make you feel red hot!

32

OVERSIZED

- **THE LOOK:** loose, natural, I-just-threw-this-on chic.

- **WEAR WITH:** leggings and jeans. Wrap a big belt round your waist to add definition to your shape, or an oversized jacket for a cool seventies *Annie Hall* take (I love that style!).

- **GOOD FIT FOR:** it's a winner for most shapes and ages – all that fabric means that you can play with proportions to suit your shape.

- **NOT THE BEST FIT FOR:** petites or skinny chicks might feel a little like *Casper the Friendly Ghost* in this look.

- **FAMOUS FOR WORKING THE LOOK:** everyone from Diane Keaton to Stella McCartney.

where to buy

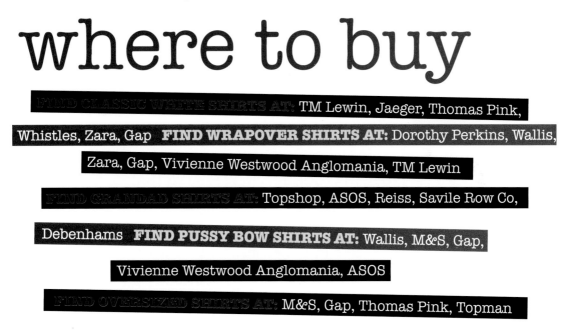

FIND CLASSIC WHITE SHIRTS AT: TM Lewin, Jaeger, Thomas Pink, Whistles, Zara, Gap **FIND WRAPOVER SHIRTS AT:** Dorothy Perkins, Wallis, Zara, Gap, Vivienne Westwood Anglomania, TM Lewin **FIND GRANDAD SHIRTS AT:** Topshop, ASOS, Reiss, Savile Row Co, Debenhams **FIND PUSSY BOW SHIRTS AT:** Wallis, M&S, Gap, Vivienne Westwood Anglomania, ASOS **FIND OVERSIZED SHIRTS AT:** M&S, Gap, Thomas Pink, Topman

SAVVY SAVER

IF YOU'VE GOT A WHITE SHIRT IN YOUR WARDROBE THAT YOU FEEL IS LOOKING A BIT THE WORSE FOR WEAR BUT WANT TO PULL OUT AGAIN, YOU CAN EASILY REVAMP IT. HERE ARE SOME TIPS ON HOW TO REFRESH IT:

1 NOW, GIRLS, I'M NOT USUALLY ONE FOR CONFORMING, BUT WHEN IT COMES TO WHITE SHIRTS, EVEN I FOLLOW THE GOLDEN RULE: it has to be as crisp and clean-looking as humanly possible. So make sure you use a good brightener: John Lewis has a great selection, and so does Dylon, which is stocked in most supermarkets.

2 THIS TIP WILL ONLY TAKE A FEW MINUTES and, even better, will only set you back about a fiver: change the buttons on your shirt for a mix of coloured ones to add designer-like detail.

3 I LOVE THAT GOOD-AS-NEW FEELING THAT DRY-CLEANED CLOTHES HAVE, but I'm not so keen on shelling out a fortune for constant trips to the dry-cleaner. Try Dr Beckmann Dry-Clean Only sheets, which you stick in the tumble-dryer for 20 minutes. What a brilliant idea! (Dr-beckmann.co.uk)

SAVVY SHOPPER

HOPEFULLY YOU'RE ALREADY WEARING YOUR FAVOURITE WHITE SHIRT IN A WHOLE NEW WAY, BUT IF YOU WANT TO START AFRESH AND BUY A NEW STYLE, HERE ARE THE DEVILISH LITTLE DETAILS TO LOOK OUT FOR:

1 WEARING GOOD FABRICS WILL MAKE OR BREAK YOUR OUTFIT, and you deserve the best, sweetheart, so always buy the best fabric you can afford – 100 per cent cotton is a pretty good benchmark. Also watch out for wonky or puffy seams and any poor finishing.

2 Now, gorgeous, the length of your shirt is so important: it can beautifully outline your shape or play havoc with it. I'd say err on the long side, as you have more fabric to play with. If your shirt is even half an inch too short, it will look and feel awkward, unless you're in a hammock in Hawaii.

3 Pay close attention to shirt necklines, girls, because the collar shape will dictate your look. Choose a round collar for a playful style. Or draw attention to your neckline with a ruffle – it will softly frame your face.

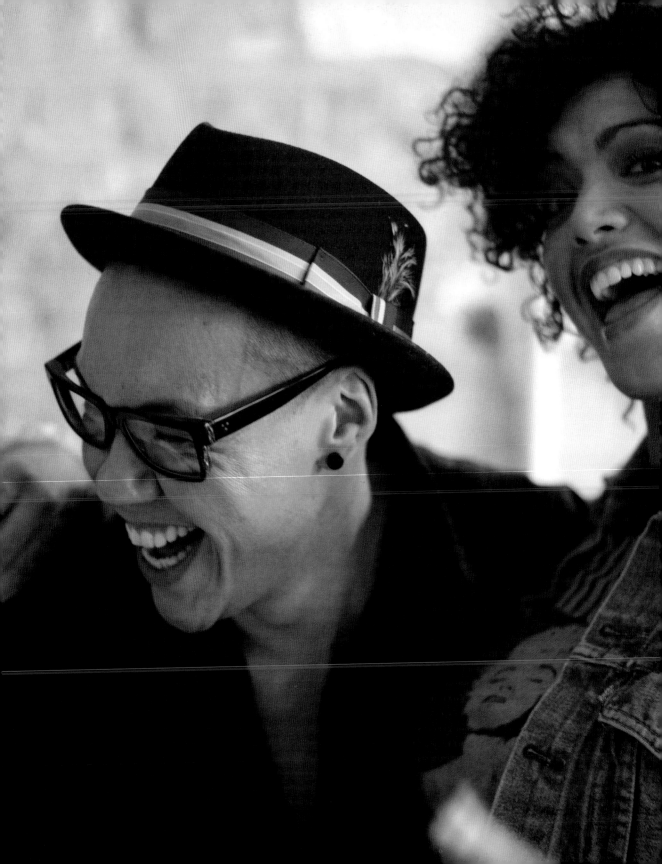

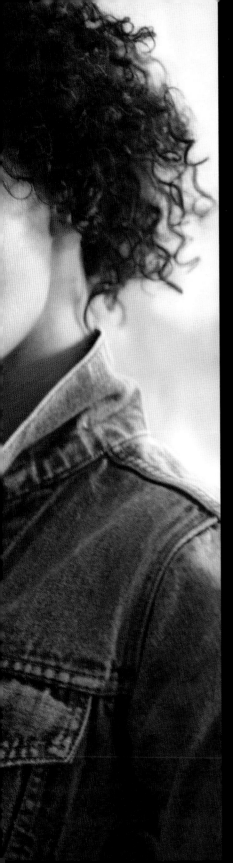

> So now you know why a white shirt is always top of the 'classic fashion' lists, ladies. I can't wait to show you how much more fashion potential this brilliant basic has in my *Timeless Style* section on page 194.

jeans

NOW, GIRLS, IF I ASKED YOU TO NAME THE TOP THREE GARMENTS that you were happy to pull out of your wardrobe every day, your jeans would be right up there at number one.

WE'VE ALL GOT A FAVOURITE PAIR THAT WE LIVE IN AND CAN'T LIVE WITHOUT; they are as comfortable as a second skin. But then jeans have always been the benchmark garment when it comes to how we feel about our bodies. On good days, your best jeans can make you feel like the sexiest person alive. On those not-so-hot days, they can make you feel anything but. And that, girls, is why we shouldn't be so quick to keep our denims in the comfy bracket – they may be the easiest thing in the world to pull on and forget about, but to get a whole lot more wear out of them, jeans need a little fashion fix, too.

Now, let's work **THREE CLASSIC JEANS STYLES** as I show you some great ways to wear them.

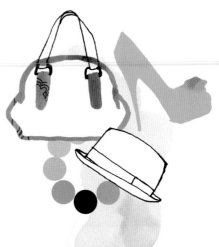

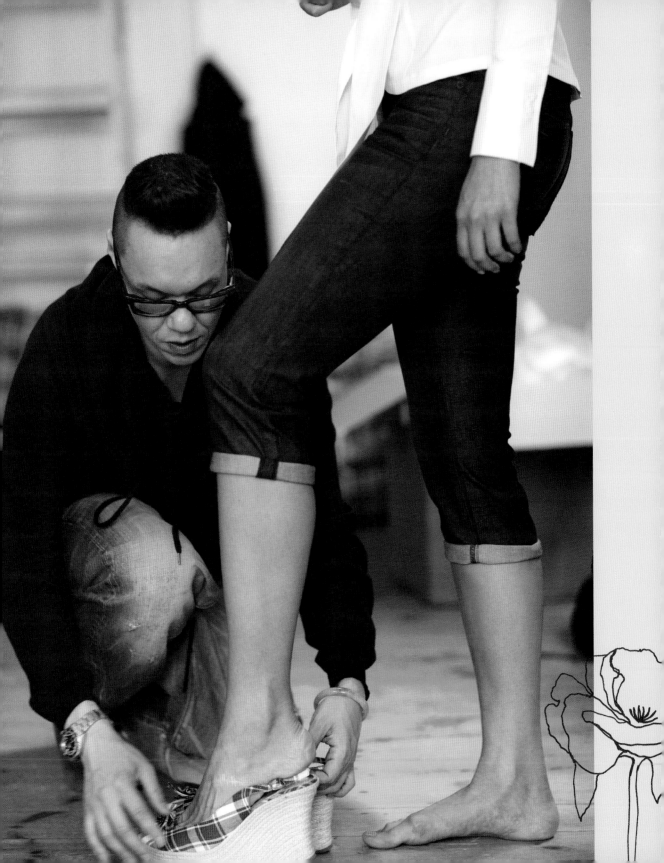

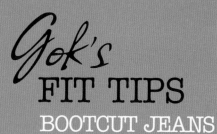

Gok's
FIT TIPS
BOOTCUT JEANS

1. Don't confuse bootcuts with flares, girls. Flares come in tight at the top of the leg and then flare out really wide at the bottom, so if you are curvy, all that fabric flapping around your ankles could make you look dumpy.

2. While a bootcut hem can perform a brilliant balancing act on pear-shaped figures, go too wide at the leg, girls, and it can make you look wide all over. (And why would you want to conceal that tiny waist!)

3. A chic, seventies-style front crease will draw the eye away from your hips and lengthen the legs.

1 *bootcut jeans*

WITH A SEXY SEVENTIES FLAVOUR, BOOTCUTS – JEANS WITH A STRAIGHT LEG THAT FLARES OUT SLIGHTLY AT THE BOTTOM – ARE ONE OF THE MOST POPULAR STYLES IN STORES NOW. They were originally designed to sit comfortably over cowboy boots, and whether down on the ranch or out on the town, bootcuts are a brilliantly versatile option for most shapes. The look? Everyday elegance is the starting point with this style, ladies. So let's make them the elegant option for you.

• SIMPLY SEXY

Jeans and T-shirts go together like summer and ice cream, and nothing says 'classic cool' more than this traditional combo. If you're tall and leggy, or perfectly petite, a plain white vest tucked into your bootcuts and finished off with a brown leather belt and some thong sandals is a uniform that

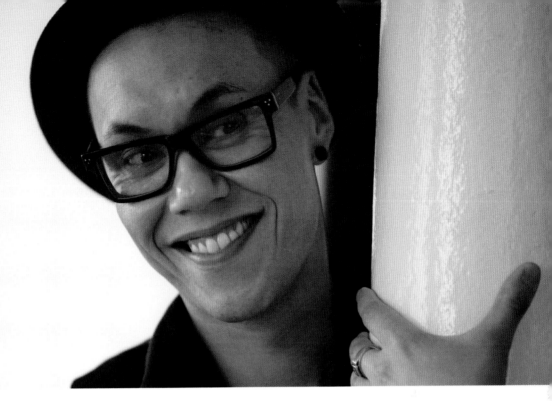

you'll want to wear every day, as it will hug your bust and curve around your shape. Other figure-flatterers include opting for a longer-length V-neck T-shirt with feminine detail, such as ruffles or puff sleeves. Choose a looser style if you are not so keen on the cling factor.

• CUTTING EDGE

I love the idea of smartening up jeans with sharp tailoring, and a neatly cut black jacket does the trick nicely. So if you are popping out for a midweek dinner date, pull out any black jacket that nips in at the waist and skims across your bottom. Styles longer than this are a no-go with bootcuts – they will turn your frame into a box, and that is certainly not hot, ladies. Roll the sleeves up and simply add heels and a slim patent belt (or any of your trusted big, sexy waist-cinchers) for added shape.

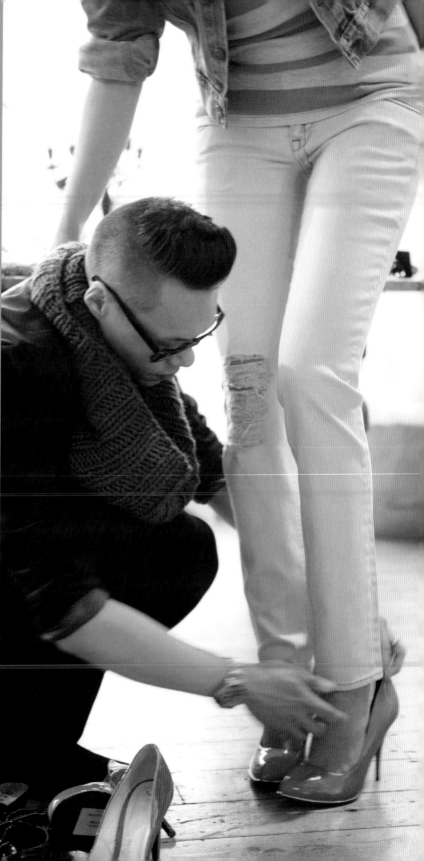

Gok's FIT TIPS
SKINNY JEANS

1. You don't have to be super-skinny to wear them, but if you feel at all uncomfortable in skinnies, be honest and go for another style.

2. I know how tempting it is to squeeze into a pair of jeans that fit you at the hips and make your legs feel like Elle Macpherson's (we've all been there, my darlings), but if they nip so tightly at the waist that your midriff hangs over them, say no to these doubtful denims.

3. Mid- to high-rise are the most flattering skinny cuts: those LA-style low-rise ones can reveal way too much. Can you hear me, Pussycat Dolls?

2 *skinny jeans*

EVERY JEANS STYLE HAS ITS OWN PERSONALITY AND SKINNIES ARE THE FUNKY ROCK CHICK OF THE GROUP. Many of the curvier girls I meet feel that skinnies are hard to pull off, but it's all about getting the balance right. If you wear a top with lots of fabric and movement, where the fabric fits under the bust and flows over your stomach and bottom, then it will even out your proportions and shape you up in no time.

• READY TO ROCK

This casual look could be known as **'THE MOSS'**, for model Kate has made that iconic rock-'n'-roll style her fashion calling card. But then Kate always gets the proportions right, and that's all you have to do to make the rock-chick look hit the right note for you. The brilliant thing about skinnies is that because your bottom half has such a neatly defined shape, you can get creative with the top. For the real rock deal, wear a big vintage print T-shirt underneath any of your jackets and loop a scarf loosely round your neck. If the colours clash, all the better, gorgeous girl.

• BEATNIK BEAUTY

This timeless look is perfect for spring or autumn days. The fact that it suits all ages, too, makes it one of my all-time favourites. If you don't like the idea of full-length super-skinnies, choose a pair that sit just above the ankle, or that have zips up the side. Pair with a stripy top, a pair of ballet flats and a classic trench coat for perfect Parisian chic. Tie a vintage silk scarf round your neck for a dash of sixties charm. Or play the casual card with a big, loose scarf. And don't forget those giant sunnies.

FIT TIPS

1. Straight legs are the classic jeans shape and will suit most figures and all ages.

2. Traditional jeans brands, such as Lee, Wrangler and Levi's, design great-quality classic straights for around £60, and because you will probably wear them for years, that's a brilliant bargain in my book.

3. If you have a beautifully boyish or petite frame, straights will give you a more defined outline.

3 *straight jeans*

THE STORY THAT YOUR STRAIGHT JEANS TELL, LADIES, IS COOL AND CLASSIC. More than most styles, straight legs never really date and are a good all-rounder. For my curvy girls who like the idea of skinny but don't want to look top-heavy, the straight is perfect for you: this style of jeans will give a leaner look and, with more depth at the crotch, a dynamic derriere, too. This classic shape is also a great bet for my older girls, as it doesn't dictate a full-on fashion look. Bring them up to date in your own natural way.

• PREP SCHOOL

In the eighties, Brooke Shields in her Calvin Kleins put designer jeans on the map. And, my darlings, regardless of your style, age or shape, in this smart-casual style, you can work a fabulous designer-denim look of your own. Just

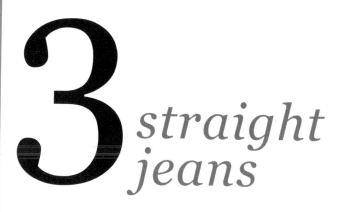

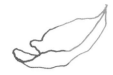

" Straight jeans will give you a leaner look and a dynamic derriere, too, gorgeous! "

whip out a casual men's-style shirt or a plain T-shirt from your wardrobe, along with a blazer. Tuck your top in and wear a tan leather belt. If you're going shopping, slip on a pair of loafers (they are so in again). Or wear courts to smarten up for a lunch date. Strings of pearls and an oversized tote will give the look that all-important 21st-century spin.

• WONDERFUL WEEKENDER

Straight jeans look fabulous when paired with an oversized batwing-sleeve jumper, and I simply adore this sexy 'I just pulled this out of the closet' look – it's a great style for all shapes. Just wear a plain vest underneath and leave the sweater to slope seductively off one shoulder. Run your fingers through your hair for that naturally sexy look. Simply gorgeous! Again, it's a look that doesn't date and will work whatever your age. Nude or natural-coloured heels are the elegant choice.

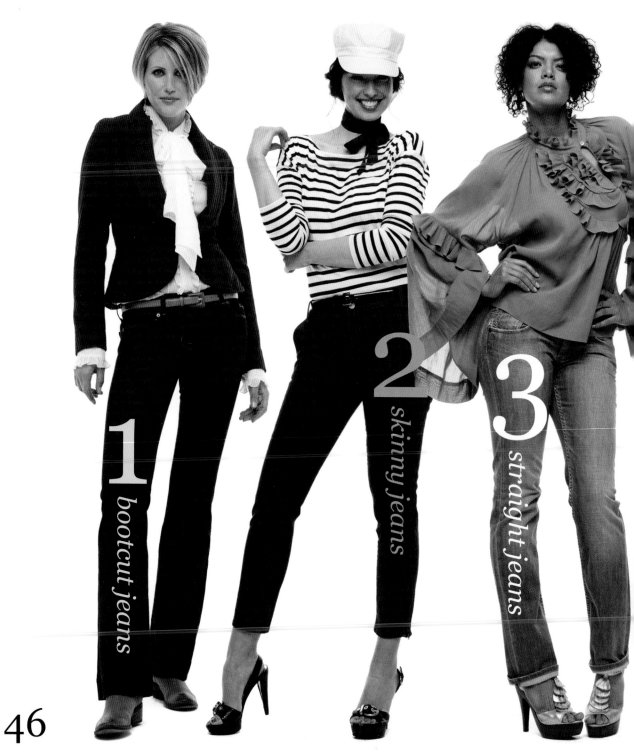

1 *bootcut jeans*

2 *skinny jeans*

3 *straight jeans*

WORK YOUR WARDROBE

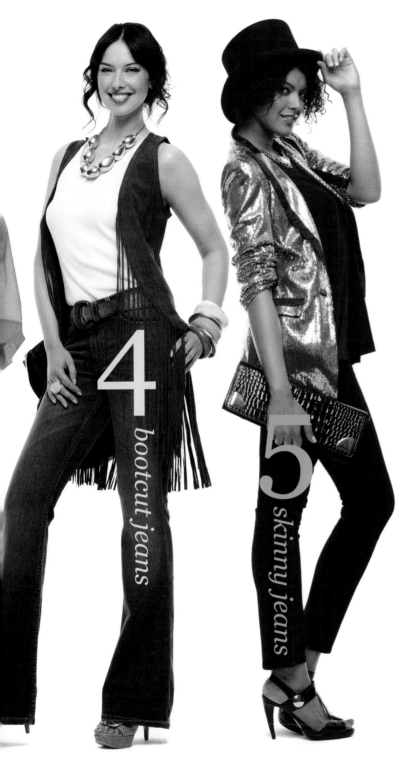

4 bootcut jeans

5 skinny jeans

> "Every jeans style has its own character – all the better to reflect yours!"

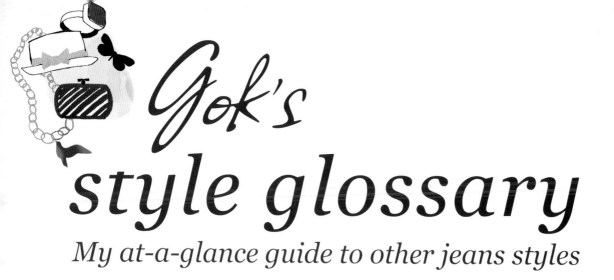

Gok's
style glossary

My at-a-glance guide to other jeans styles

THE BOYFRIEND

- **THE LOOK:** just-thrown-together cool. Low-slung at the waist and baggy at the legs – roll up these casual denims just above the ankle and wear with heels for a girlie boyfriend look.

- **WEAR WITH:** a loose boyfriend shirt and platform heels, or a stripy T-shirt and plimsolls or pumps.

- **GOOD FIT FOR:** girls with slimmer thighs and boyish frames.

- **NOT THE BEST FIT FOR:** curvy or tall girls.

- **FAMOUS FOR WORKING THE LOOK:** Katie Holmes.

THE HIGH-WAISTED FLARE

- **THE LOOK:** this oh-so-seventies style is cut high above the waist with a very wide flare at the hem.

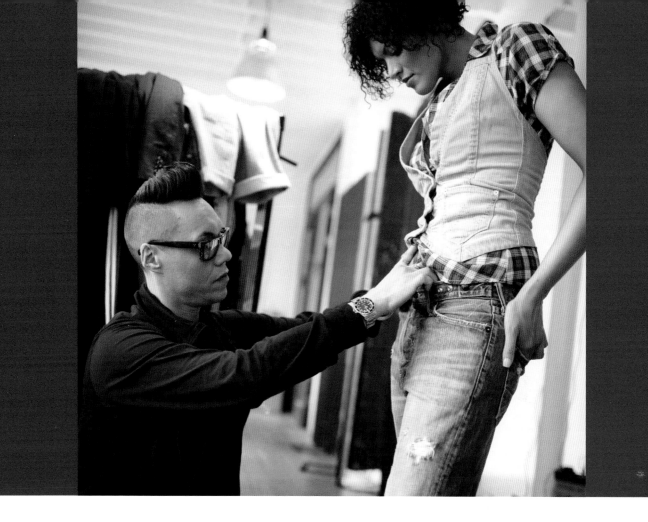

- **WEAR WITH:** tight-fitting T-shirts and lots of long, gold necklaces. Wedge sandals will finish off the look.

- **GOOD FIT FOR:** petites (but don't go too wide on the flare) and boyish figures. Button-front ones are good for flattering tummies.

- **NOT THE BEST FIT FOR:** hourglass shapes or curvy girls.

- **FAMOUS FOR WORKING THE LOOK:** Cheryl Cole.

Gok's denim checklist

Make sure your denims are ticking all the right boxes with a little extra style know-how.

1. JEANS GENIUS?

Please, please, ladies, when it comes to buying jeans, do not be bullied by the size on the label. Jeans will only look truly fabulous if they fit. You deserve to look amazing in your jeans, and the better the fit, the better you'll look.

2. THE STRETCH FACTOR

Too much elastic can make your jeans stretch an inch too far, especially around the waist and bum area. My advice? Take a good look at the label: any jeans with 2 per cent elastane or under will be a good fit and keep your jeans – and you – looking red hot, honey!

3. DEDICATED FOLLOWER

When it comes to jeans, your body has to tell you what's in – not fashion magazines and not current trends. If CHERYL COLE is doing flared jeans, then let Cheryl go off and do them: they are brilliant for her shape. You, my darlings, have to find the jeans that are brilliant for yours.

4. ON THE RISE

The balance between the waist and the crotch is known as the 'rise'. Here's my quick guide: low-rise waistbands sit a few inches below your belly button; medium or regular rises sit just underneath it; and high rises are cut just above.

5. POCKET POWER

Pay close attention to pockets, ladies: they can make a phenomenal difference in the derriere department. If you want to create a curvy J-Lo effect (and who wouldn't?), look for jeans with a button-down pocket, as they will 'lift' your behind. Pocket seams that draw down into a point will give added definition to the buttocks and so are good for bootylicious babes. Bigger pockets are also a good butt-balancer for you.

6. WORK IT

We are so relaxed about dress codes now that it's not unusual to wear jeans to work. But even if it's a dress-down day, why not keep up the glam factor? Treat dress-down days as a dress-up treat – a chance to wear what you like in your own special way. They may cost a little more, but smart, tailored jeans in dark washes can look knockout in the office.

7. LENGTHY BUSINESS

Whether you are wearing stilettos or flats, the hem on your jeans should cover your ankles and skim just above the heel. If the hems are too long, you can look as though you have wheels rather than feet – there needs to be a distinction between the hem and your foot.

8. A MATTER OF CHOICE

We all have two personalities – I've got Downtown Gok and Uptown Gok – and so it is with jeans: if you are a denim diva and they are the essence of your style, I'd recommend that you have two pairs in your wardrobe. Yes, we all have faves that we love to dress up and dress down, but you don't want to wear one pair to death. Think about getting two pairs in different cuts.

9. TO BOLDLY GO

From raspberry to super-faded and black to brilliant white, different colours and washes can add a fresh twist. White jeans are just such a fabulous basic and have a great uptown-chic feel, whether rock-chick skinny or sailor-pant style. Watch out for bleached-out patches on the fronts of jeans, though: they can be horribly unflattering. Pale washes can make your legs look big, too – an optical illusion I'm sure we would all be happy to avoid.

10. DOUBLE D

A top-to-toe denim and cowboy boot look can be a bit BUTCH CASSIDY for my liking, unless, of course, you want to look like an extra from *Dallas* (and I'm not talking Pammy – that all-denim look is more ranch-hand chic than eighties chick). Instead, break up the blue with a pretty top, shoes or accessories.

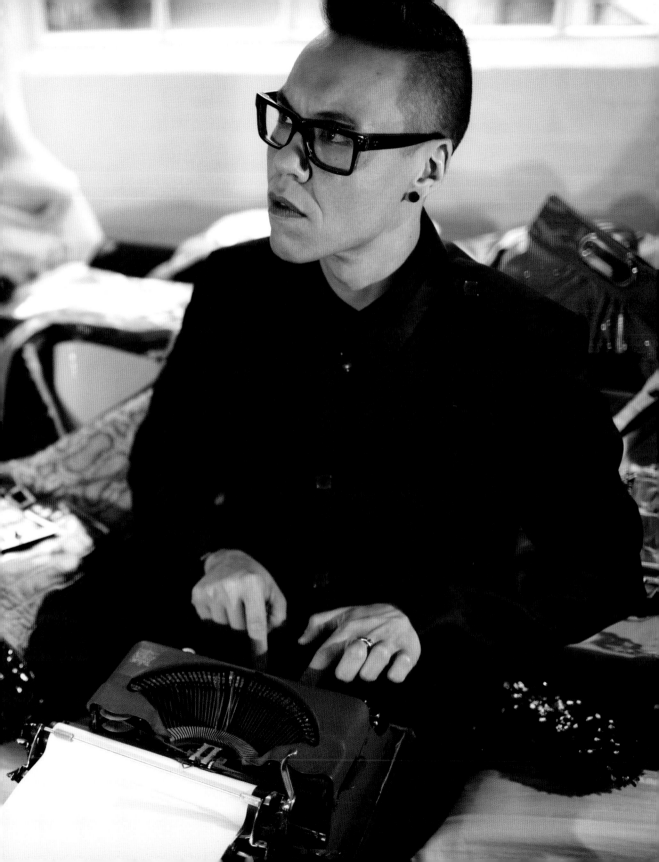

SAVVY SAVER

THE BRILLIANT THING ABOUT JEANS, ANGELS, IS THAT YOU CAN WEAR THE SAME OLD PAIR FOR YEARS. ALL IT TAKES IS A LITTLE STYLE KNOW-HOW TO GIVE THEM AN INSTANT UPDATE.

1 ALTERATIONS, ALTERATIONS, ALTERATIONS! They're a fashionista's best friend. It's tempting just to stick with hems at the length they were when you bought them, or to leave legs bagging round the thighs because they fit you at the waist, but jeans alterations usually only cost a few quid and I can't tell you how much they will ramp up the revamp factor.

2 THE WAR IS OVER, GIRLS, SO THERE'S NO NEED TO BOIL-WASH YOUR DENIMS TO DEATH. Keep your jeans looking better for longer: wash them at 40 degrees. Also, turn them inside out before you put them in the machine.

3 CHARITY BEGINS AT HOME AND WHEN IT COMES TO GREAT-PRICED DENIMS, second-hand shops are a godsend. When I'm styling, charity shops are one of my first ports of call, because the denim selections are fabulous – not to mention fabulously well priced. Have a good rummage and you're sure to find some fab styles.

SAVVY SHOPPER

SHOPPING FOR JEANS CAN BE A TOUGH CALL THESE DAYS – YOU NEED A MAP TO NAVIGATE ALL THE STYLES AND CUTS ON OFFER. SO HERE ARE MY SIMPLE POINTERS TO SET YOU ON YOUR WAY TO FINDING THE PERFECT PAIR.

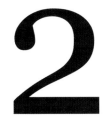

1 MAKE **GAP** YOUR FIRST STOP: they have really cut to the chase with the way they label their jeans and have made it so easy to recognise which shape is which.

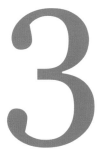

2 THE PRICES OF SOME DENIMS ARE REACHING LEVELS THAT WOULD MAKE A HOLLYWOOD HEIRESS THINK TWICE. Yes, I know that some are beautifully cut, so if you have the cash to splash on a special pair, then treat yourself. But I think traditional brands, such as Wrangler, Lee and Levi's, give you as much for your money – after all, they have been making jeans for centuries.

3 IF YOU ARE GOING JEANS SHOPPING, MAKE SURE YOU HAVE A PAIR OF HEELS WITH YOU, and try to fit a fave top in your bag, too. It really helps to style jeans up before you buy. Plus, having some of your other key pieces to hand will encourage you to try new styles.

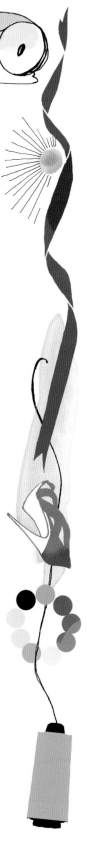

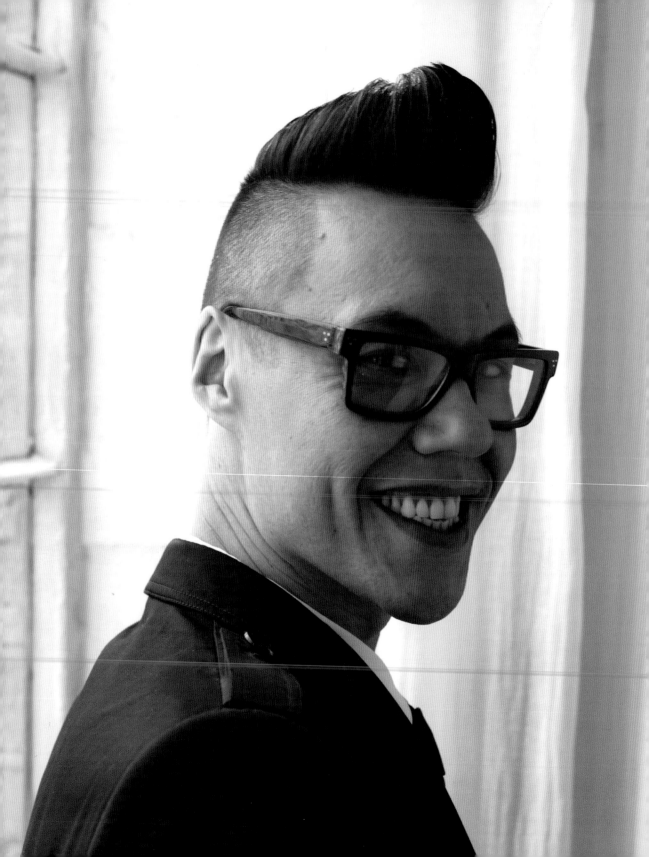

where to buy

FIND BOOTCUT JEANS AT: Wrangler, Topshop, Gap, John Lewis, M&S, House of Fraser **FIND SKINNY JEANS AT:** Topshop, Uniqlo, ASOS, River Island, Diesel **FIND STRAIGHT JEANS AT:** Levi's stores, high-street jeans specialists (for Levi's, Wrangler and Lee), House of Fraser (for mid-range designer), Ilovejeans.com **FIND BOYFRIEND JEANS AT:** Dorothy Perkins, Gap, New Look **FIND HIGH-WAISTED FLARES AT:** French Connection, Topshop, ASOS

66

So now you know how the jeans that you wear every day can be easily styled to make you feel fabulous, whatever your mood.

99

trousers

TROUSER SHAPES HAVE REALLY CHANGED OVER THE PAST COUPLE OF YEARS, with designers offering us everything from the peg leg to the harem pant and the spray-on skinny.

WHILE I AM A GREAT BELIEVER IN TRYING OUT NEW SHAPES (it's a great first step to refreshing your style, girls), I think there's so much fashion potential in classic styles that you don't have to rush out and buy the latest trouser trends every season – phew! That's not to say that finding even a classic pair to suit your shape is an easy task; many of my ladies say that they find trouser shopping tricky. But if you do have a pair, those timeless trousers should be the brilliant back-up to your little black dress: a dependable, do-all closet classic that will suit you from day to night, desk to dancefloor and beyond.

Now, my angels, let's take a look at some of the **CLASSIC TROUSER STYLES** that I find hanging up in most of my girls' wardrobes.

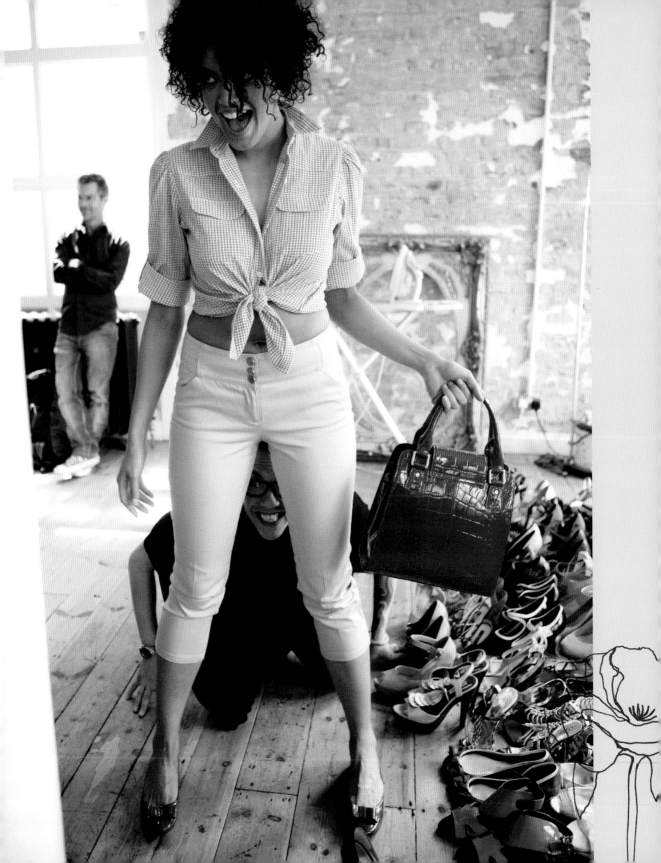

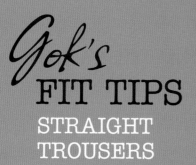

Gok's
FIT TIPS
STRAIGHT TROUSERS

1. Flat-fronted straights will work wonders on my girls who prefer to keep their midriff under wraps, as they can streamline the tummy area.

2. Defined front seams will elongate straight legs, but juicy girls beware: if the seams stretch and flatten across the hips, it can focus attention on this area.

3. Pinstripe trousers can do wonders for curvy shapes by drawing the eye right round them. They can also make legs look longer.

1 *straight trousers*

WHEN IT COMES TO TAILORED BLACK TROUSERS, STRAIGHT LEGS CAN REALLY LENGTHEN THOSE PINS, SO WHAT'S NOT TO LOVE? Straight doesn't necessarily mean straightforward, though, and because there are quite a few different options, it's worth looking at whether the ones you wear are working well for you. As is always the way, ladies, when making your classic pieces work to suit your shape, it all comes down to detail. So check the waistband and leg style (straight cuts vary slightly in width), and follow my 'Fit Tips' for the best straights to suit your shape.

• CITY SLICKER

It doesn't take long to make these simple staples into a super-stylish office get-up, whatever your age or shape. Just pair with a plain black fitted shirt, add a classic black or tan belt with a smart metal buckle (gold or silver will work) to define the waist, slip on a pair of statement flats (pumps with jewels or buckles on) and hang a classic black jacket casually over your shoulders for that ever-elegant European chic. Or, for a sharper look, slip on a sumptuously silky vest top (wear a slouchy fine-knit cardie over that if you don't like the tops of your arms on show), turn up your trousers to the ankle and slip on some power heels. Accessorise with a scarf or necklaces. Whichever route you choose, darling divas, style central is your destination.

• BLACK NIGHTS

When it comes to dressing for evening or putting together an easy office-to-party look, black slim pants are the wings of any social butterfly. To make your work trousers say 'fashion-week chic', just slip on one of your black silky blouses and wrap a super-wide belt (at least 6 inches) between the waistband of your trousers and your bust. A sequined belt or a classic cummerbund will do. (I always find them in charity shops.) No one will ever know you are wearing your work trousers, while the wide belt will elongate your mid-section beautifully. Just kick off your flats, jump into your heels and you've given these pants a super-sultry evening spin.

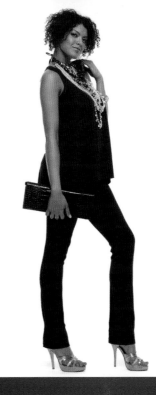

"

Kick off your flats, jump into your heels and you've given these pants a super-sultry evening spin.

"

61

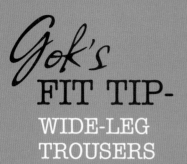

Gok's FIT TIP-
WIDE-LEG TROUSERS

1. Watch out for pleating and drawstring styles, as they can add bulk to your tummy.

2. Wide pants will work wonders on my lovely pear-shaped girls, especially if the trouser waistline is ever so slightly high.

3. Wide pants are a great option for my older girls – they say smart, sophisticated and just the right side of sexy.

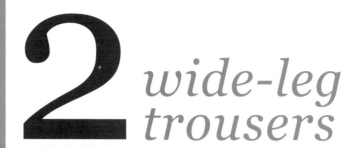

2 *wide-leg trousers*

NOTHING SAYS OLD-STYLE GLAMOUR LIKE WIDE-LEG PANTS: THEY NEVER, EVER DATE. They can be worn at any age and just ooze the kind of easy elegance that says, 'effortless glamour'. They appear on the catwalks every season and have earned their status as a classic style statement. Whether high-waisted low-slung pyjama pants or tailored fit and flare, they can speak volumes about your style. But, ladies, there is one absolutely crucial style tip when it comes to wide pants: they should never be a millimetre too short. Ultimately, they should skim the bottom of your heel (without trailing). Hems shorter than this will shorten your frame, too.

• THE SLOUCH
This casual-chic option is a great choice for all my sexy slims, leggy lovelies or pear-shaped beauties. With its long, flowing feel, this pyjama-pant style is perfect for summer parties, or for promenading

along the beachfront in sunnier climes. The best wide cuts for this are flat-fronted styles with side pockets. Wear with a fitted top – a simple vest is the perfect partner (a stripy twin set would also look the business), then pile on big chunky bangles up your wrists for contemporary Chanel-style chic.

• NIGHT MOVES

No one does shimmering wide pants better than Giorgio Armani; the Italian designer pretty much invented this super-sophisticated take on occasion dressing. But, girls, you don't need a designer budget to carry this look off. Just keep it simple by layering clothes in luxurious fabrics and neutral tones (all black, or varied shades of grey, for instance). So if you are wearing plain black trousers, choose a black top with a bit of sparkle about it – a sequin-sprinkled vest, for instance – pile on necklaces, bracelets and earrings in the same shade and slip on a black jacket. Or dare to bare and just wear a pretty lace-trim camisole under the jacket.

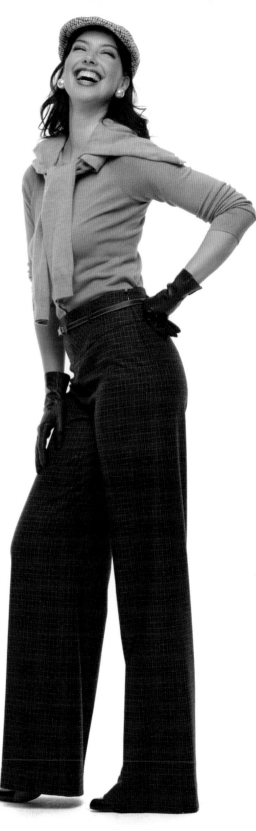

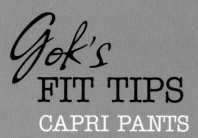

Gok's
FIT TIPS
CAPRI PANTS

1. Beware cropped trousers with a wide hem – they can make you look like a pirate in search of a ship.

2. Wear heels for a more contemporary capri look; they will make your legs look long and slim, too.

3. Capris are great for my tummy-shy girls – they make the most of your shapely legs.

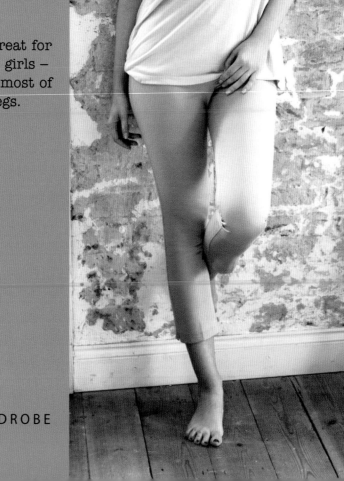

64

3 *capri pants*

AUDREY HEPBURN DID AS MUCH FOR THE CLASSIC CAPRI-PANT LOOK as she did for the little black dress. Her cropped trousers, crew-neck sweater and ballet pumps combo is a look that still hits the right note with all you sexy stylistas. But capri pants have been constantly updated since Audrey made them a fashion hit, meaning that every year there are more options to help you make this short and sweet classic a fashion hit for you.

• DAY TO DAY

For a simple take on that sensational fifties St Tropez look, simply pick a checked – or gingham – shirt out of your wardrobe and play around with belts to get the right style for your shape. Add a pair of ballet pumps, a gorgeous shopper and your most over-the-top sunnies for a day out with the girls. Or opt for a leggier, sexier look with some towering wedges. If the weather is more Morecambe Bay than St Tropez, sling a mac on top!

• DRESS IT UP

Because they are such a slim shape, capris are great for adding layers to. And for night, you don't always have to stick to darker shades. I love sand-coloured crop pants worn with a top in a similarly soft shade. I'd play with the proportions by wearing a big, baggy blouse or top, or one with voluminous sleeves. Then, my lovelies, you can just accessorise away: an oversized necklace and bangles in a starkly contrasting colour will add drama.

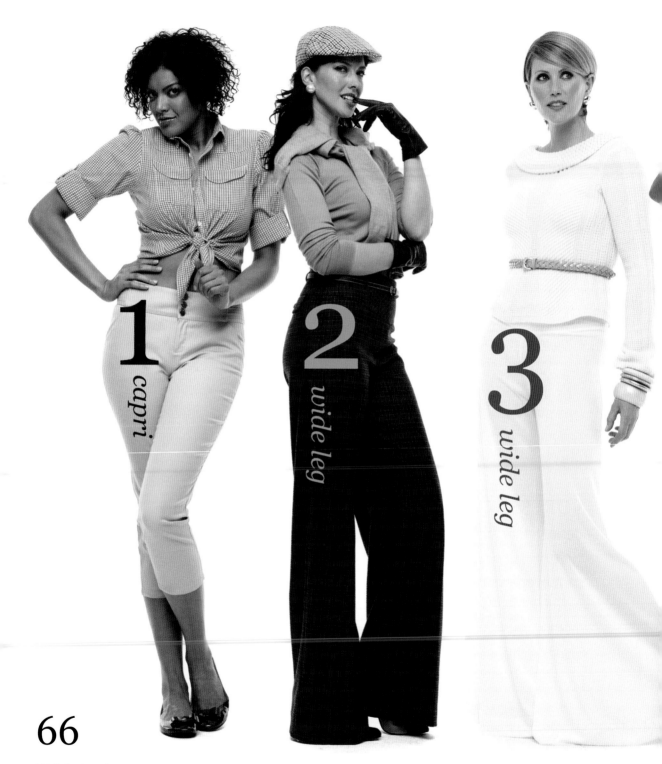

1 *capri*

2 *wide leg*

3 *wide leg*

WORK YOUR WARDROBE

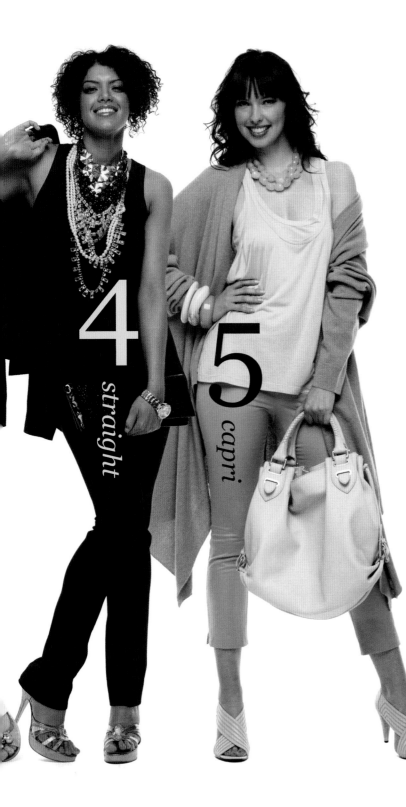

4 *straight*

5 *capri*

> "Classic trousers can be a great back-up to your little black dress."

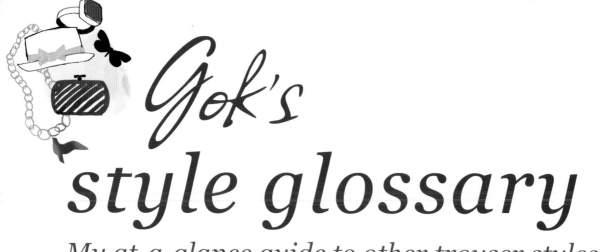

Gok's
style glossary

My at-a-glance guide to other trouser styles

THE CHINO

- **THE LOOK:** these loose, casual, pleat-front cotton trousers are the last word in sporty, preppy chic.

- **WEAR WITH:** a big slouchy top (wear loose to cover the tummy, or tucked in if you're petite or slim), or plain vests and T-shirts. Roll up to the ankle and slip on some ballet pumps or sandals. Wear heels if you want to balance out your hips or bottom.

- **GOOD FIT FOR:** slim, boyish figures.

- **NOT THE BEST FIT FOR:** curvy girls.

- **FAMOUS FOR WORKING THE LOOK:** Kylie Minogue.

THE PEG

- **THE LOOK:** these casual cotton trousers are usually big and baggy at the waistband and hips, then taper down to the

68

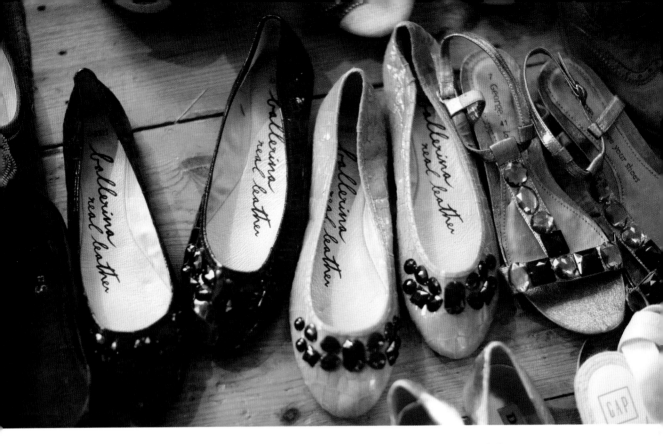

ankle. They epitomise that notion of smart-casual dressing.

- **WEAR WITH:** a crisp white shirt or vest and a waistcoat (always tuck tops in to pegs as you need to see the waist detail), or a mannish blazer and towering heels.

- **GOOD FIT FOR:** straight-up-and-down girls and slim chicks.

- **NOT THE BEST FIT FOR:** pretty pears (the tapered leg will highlight your hips) and curvy girls (the pleating round the waist could add extra inches here, too).

- **FAMOUS FOR WORKING THE LOOK:** Keira Knightley.

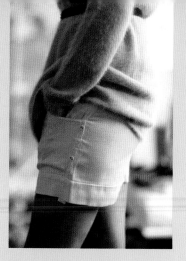

A little word about ...
SHORTS

DON'T WAIT FOR SUNNY DAYS TO WHIP SHORTS OUT OF THE WARDROBE: when worn with opaque tights, shorts can look just as sassy in the autumn months as they do in summer. One of my favourite looks is the city short. Because they are tailored, city shorts can have a real slimming effect on most figures. And if some of my **OLDER GIRLS** don't like the idea of wearing them to work, looser casual styles are a great weekender option. In summer, wear them with a white cotton blouse. (Keep it loose if your stomach is more wobbly than washboard.) **CURVY GIRLS**, keep your top half cinched in at the waist to highlight that hot hourglass shape. **PETITES**, go for tailored on top, too. (Your basic white shirt, tucked in, would be a nice, neat style for you.) Wear heels for a sexy touch, or wow with wedges – they look great with shorts in summer. But, my gorgeous girls, leave the plimsolls in the porch: they'll say 'ship ahoy' more than shipshape. If you are a whiter-than-white angel, smooth a little fake tan on to your pins for a heavenly golden glow.

A little word about ...
TROUSER SUITS

IN THE EARLY SEVENTIES, FRENCH FASHION DESIGNER YVES SAINT LAURENT BECAME FAMOUS FOR TURNING THE TRADITIONAL MEN'S TROUSER SUIT INTO A SUPER-SEXY OPTION FOR WOMEN and it's a look that I think women still look amazing in today. Often designed in traditional men's pinstripe fabric, YSL's suits were such a hit because they were cut to show off women's figures: so jackets came in sharply at the waist, while the trousers were long and slim on the hip and flared out a little at the bottom. And, my angels, these are just the key points to look out for when wearing trouser suits today. You can also up the feminine factor by wearing a gloriously girlie blouse – your pussy bow would work wonders here. Just add some high, high heels. **Gorgeous!**

SAVVY SAVER

YOUR FAVE TROUSERS CAN EASILY BE GIVEN A NEW LEASE OF LIFE. HERE'S HOW:

1 PULL OUT ALL THE TROUSERS THAT YOU HAVE HANGING UP IN YOUR WARDROBE (and, yes, that means those sale bargains that you bought last year that still have the label on!) and sort them into two piles: the ones that you will wear again and those that you just never want to put on. Now, pack the second pile off to the charity shop or to a car-boot sale. Then look at the ones you have left with a fresh eye and consider new ways to wear them.

2 FEELING A LITTLE BORED WITH YOUR EVERYDAY TROUSERS, GIRLS? Then completely change their look with some simple alterations: transform bootcuts into straights by tapering them in from the knee down: just ask a girlfriend to help you pin them. Take them to be altered or, if you're handy with a machine, DIY!

3 YOU TOO CAN GET THAT YVES SAINT LAURENT LOOK WITH A LITTLE DESIGNER KNOW-HOW: just take a pair of plain black trousers (straight or wide) and stitch a strip of black velvet ribbon (go as thick or as thin as you like, ladies) down the side seams of each trouser leg for a glamorous evening 'tux' look.

SAVVY SHOPPER

SWOT UP ON YOUR TROUSER KNOW-HOW BEFORE YOU HIT
THE SHOPS, LADIES:

1 IF YOU FIND A PAIR OF TROUSERS THAT ARE A PERFECT FIT
ROUND THE WAIST BUT A BIT BIGGLES-LIKE ON THE HIPS, THEN
CONSIDER HAVING THEM TAKEN IN – a little bit of DIY tailoring
can give that made-to-measure edge at a fraction of the price.

2 TAKE DIFFERENT TOPS INTO THE CHANGING
ROOM WHEN YOU ARE SHOPPING FOR TROUSERS.
It will help you picture a whole load of looks and
give you an idea of how they will work with some
of the jackets and tops you already have hanging
in your wardrobe.

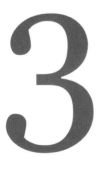

3 IF YOU WEAR TROUSERS A LOT, I'D SUGGEST GOING ONE
STEP UP FROM MAINSTREAM HIGH STREET LABELS AND
SPLASHING A LITTLE MORE CASH ON A WELL-TAILORED
PAIR IN A GOOD FABRIC. Boutiques such as Whistles,
Jigsaw, Reiss and Jaeger are the places to search for these
styles. You may have to spend a little more but your
trousers will look good as new – and on-trend – for years
to come.

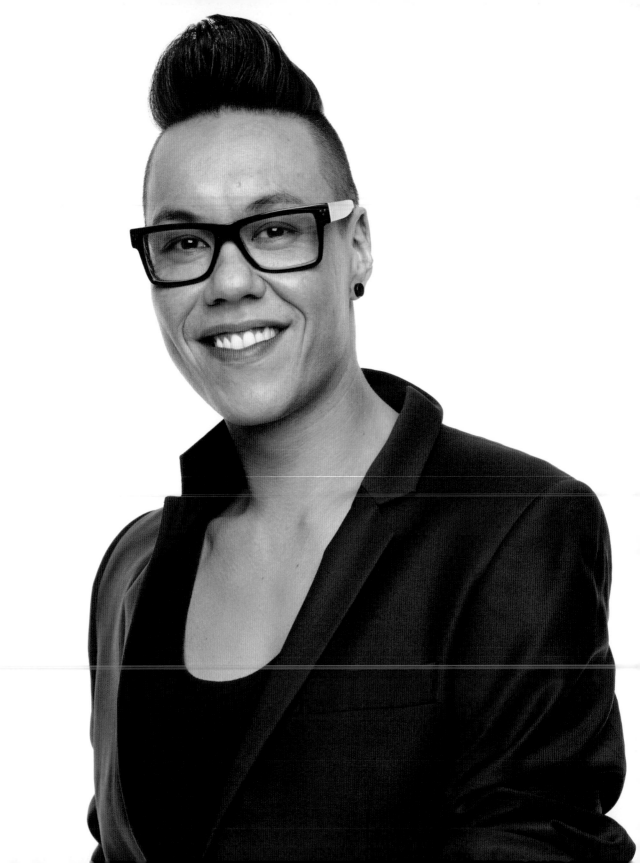

where to buy

FIND STRAIGHT TROUSERS AT: Gap, French Connection, Diesel

FIND WIDE-LEG TROUSERS AT: Zara, Jaeger, H&M **FIND CAPRI PANTS**

AT: Topshop, Uniqlo, Gap, M&S **FIND CHINOS AT:** Gap, Levi's,

French Connection **FIND PEGS AT:** Reiss, Topshop, Whistles

66

Now you know why you don't need a designer budget to get a lot more wear out of your trousers, girls. For other ways to wear them, check out my *Timeless Style* section on page 194.

99

tops

WHENEVER I DELVE INTO MY GORGEOUS GIRLS' WARDROBES, I'M ALWAYS AMAZED AT THE AMOUNT OF CLOTHES THEY HAVE CRAMMED IN THERE THAT THEY ADMIT TO NEVER WEARING. And not only are tops the biggest offenders on the 'never been worn' pile, they always come top of the 'can't decide which to wear' list.

THE REASON FOR THESE CLOTHING CONUNDRUMS, YOU NAUGHTY HOARDERS, IS THAT YOU HAVE TOO MUCH CHOICE. The only way to avert this clothing crisis is to delve into that Tardis of tops and be ruthless about the ones you love and those you really loathe. To give you a head start, I've highlighted a handful of classic styles that are likely to be hanging up in your wardrobe. By styling them up and sharing my tips on how to get the most out of your tops, I'll show you how keeping things simple will streamline your wardrobe and sass up your style.

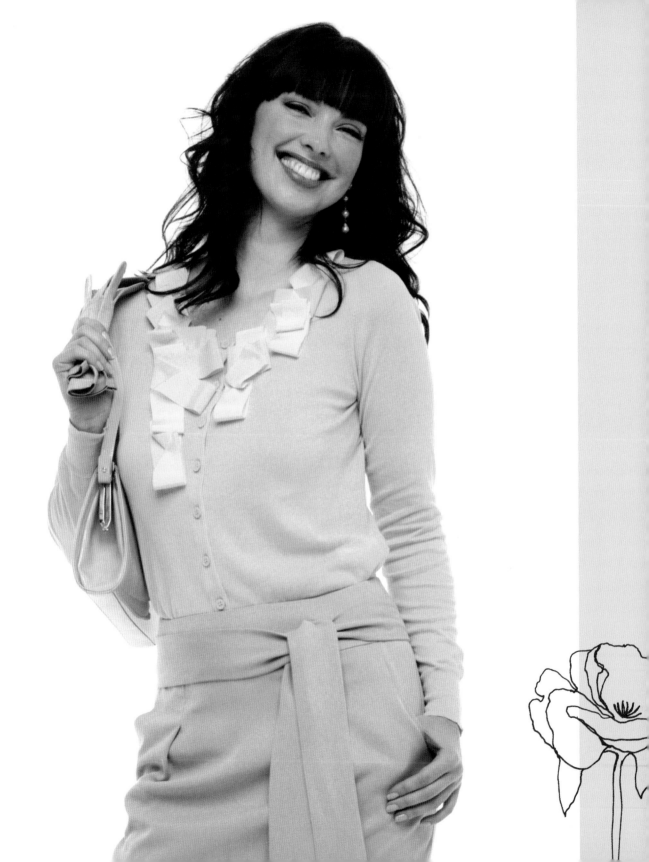

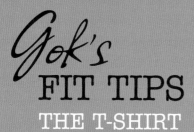

Gok's
FIT TIPS
THE T-SHIRT

1. Unless you're a teenager, bargain vest tops are great for layering under shirts and cardies, but they can bare a bit too much flesh when worn on their own with bra straps showing through.

2. If your tummy is your trouble spot, traditional T-shirt shapes are not the ideal fit for you as they will tend to cling around the middle. Instead, go for looser, slouchier styles that gather in a band under the tummy.

3. White T-shirts show every lump and bump: loose, white cotton shirts are a more flattering option for curvier girls.

1 *the T-shirt*

T-SHIRTS ARE THE BACKBONE OF MANY A WARDROBE, AND, LIKE OUR FAVOURITE JEANS, THEY ARE JUST SO EASY TO PULL ON AND FORGET ABOUT. Take it from me, though, girls, it's worth remembering that your T-shirt can make or break an outfit, and if yours is to fall into the 'make-it' category, you need to think outside the straight T-shape: go for slouchy vests and fitted tees. (Check that your T-shirt curves in at the waist, otherwise it can look too blocky and stocky.) The good news is that there are so many styles of tees out there now that you shouldn't have any problem finding a fabulous fit. By using the simple vest as an example, I'm going to show you how easy it is to turn this staple into statement in a few easy steps.

• SIMPLY SENSATIONAL

There are so many vest variations – from plain cotton to ribbed, silky and slouchy – that you can create a whole wardrobe of different looks from them. Your vest is also the perfect undergarment, as it's not too bulky, is easy to layer up and comes in varying lengths, so you can always find one that suits your shape and style. My favourite way to dress up a vest is to balance the plain top with a more detailed bottom. So, for day, why not pair yours with a pencil skirt and a big, glam statement belt, or work it with a pair of statement trousers, such as silky harem or printed palazzo pants. Bold ethnic-style jewellery and bangles also look brilliant against a simple vest backdrop.

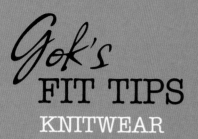

Gok's
FIT TIPS
KNITWEAR

1. V-neck knits are great for most body shapes. Some people say that if you have a flat chest you can't do them, but I think that's rubbish. You might not have shapely boobs, but you are just as sexy. V-necks give an elegant look to your top half and show off just the right amount of skin.

2. Crew-neck sweaters or T-shirts will always give your outfit a classic preppy twist. Layer up with scarves for added style.

3. Belted cardies can look great, but, ladies, I'd advise against wearing thicker belts as they can look bulky.

2 *the* *cardigan*

IT USED TO BE SEEN AS THE NORA BATTY OF FASHION – good for ramping up the frump factor and not much else – but the humble cardie (in fact, knitwear in general) has seen a real style renaissance over the past few years, with designers giving it pride of place in both their summer and winter collections. No wonder: you can really play around when you are styling up knits, which means it's easier to make them flatter your shape. So, with a little style know-how, you can go from prim and pretty to cool and contemporary. Now, let's reach into those wardrobes and revamp those long-neglected knits. Here are some ideas to get you started.

• TOUGH LOVE

It's long been hailed as one of the staples of any capsule wardrobe, but the twinset is tricky to pull off. In order to offset any primness, you really need to toughen it up. So tuck the sweater into a pair of

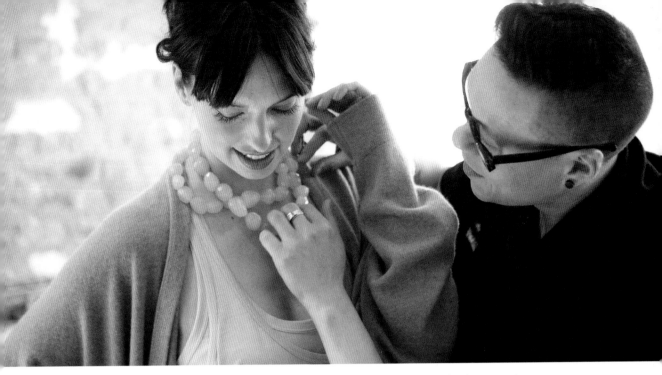

high-waisted trousers, button down the cardie to just above the bust and give it a sharper edge with a thin studded belt. Alternatively, if you like a touch of tradition, vamp up your twin-set top with a statement collar necklace or piles and piles of short-strand pearls. A pair of statement heels will add an edgier feel.

• LONG STORY

Longer-length – or boyfriend – cardigans are really hot just now, with labels such as **BURBERRY** and **STELLA McCARTNEY** giving them new classic status. A long-length cardie is a brilliant garment for any shape, and whether you want to play down your wobbly bits or concentrate on your curves, there's a lot you can do with it. I like it simply belted over a vest (try more than one belt for a chic look). If you've got great pins, you can do the whole eighties thing and wear you cardi with a pair of skinnies and stilettos, sexy girl.

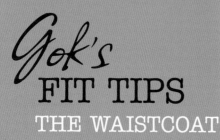

1. Outsized or mannish waistcoats look best worn loose. For a sharper look, choose one that comes in at the waist.

2. Really expose the V-shape at the neck of your waistcoat, as it will bring your shape in and out at all your best points.

3. Look for shorter, looser styles and different fabrics to suit your shape. Your waistcoat doesn't have to be a traditional suit style.

3 *the waistcoat*

OK, LADIES, I HAVE TO ADMIT THAT I AM ADDICTED TO WAISTCOATS – I HAVE ABOUT 40 OF THEM IN MY WARDROBE – AND I SERIOUSLY RECOMMEND THAT YOU START STOCKPILING THIS WARDROBE WONDER, TOO.

Believe me, girls, if you are having a bad tummy day, just bang on a waistcoat: it will work with your shape and mould itself to your body, pulling you in at the waist beautifully, while flattening you out at the front. I guarantee that its sensational structure will make you feel sensational too. The waistcoat's classic credentials mean that it can be worn at any age and styled up for most shapes. Whether it's cropped or long, denim or traditional three-piece-suit style, there are so many ways to work it into your look. **HERE'S HOW:**

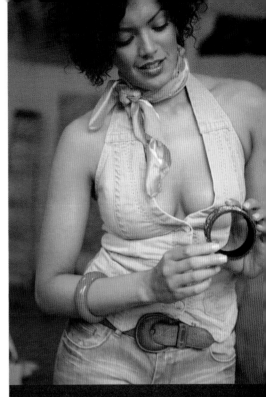

• CASUAL COOL

I love the way that waistcoats can instantly lift a relaxed look – the tailored lines really add style confidence to classic casual get-ups, such as denims and a white shirt – and that's exactly what I would do here: slip your waistcoat on top of a shirt, blouse or tee and pair it with your favourite jeans. A chunky leather (or plaited) belt, some statement heels (or tuck your jeans into square-heeled boots) and a mini shoulder bag will add a hint of Dallas-style glam to your look. If it's summer, layer your waistcoat over some different-length fine-cotton tees. Bang on some big bangles and earrings to add interest.

• SUMMER SMART

If you have a traditional waistcoat in your wardrobe (perhaps it's part of a work suit), then you can loosen it up for a chic summer look by either pairing it with a casual white shirt or wearing it over a floral, ruffle or girlie dress. Just slip on some gladiator sandals for flirty festival chic. Or, for evening, wear your waistcoat over a tailored high-collar white shirt and pair it with a pencil skirt. A long, medallion-style necklace or strings of pearls will switch on the 'now' factor.

66

A chunky leather belt will add some Dallas-style glam to your look.

99

83

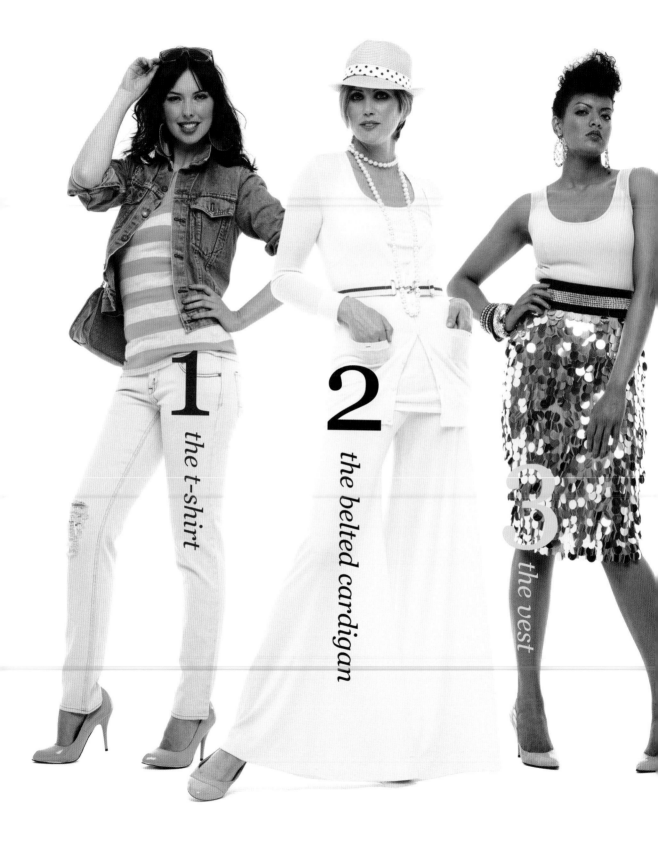

1 *the t-shirt*

2 *the belted cardigan*

3 *the vest*

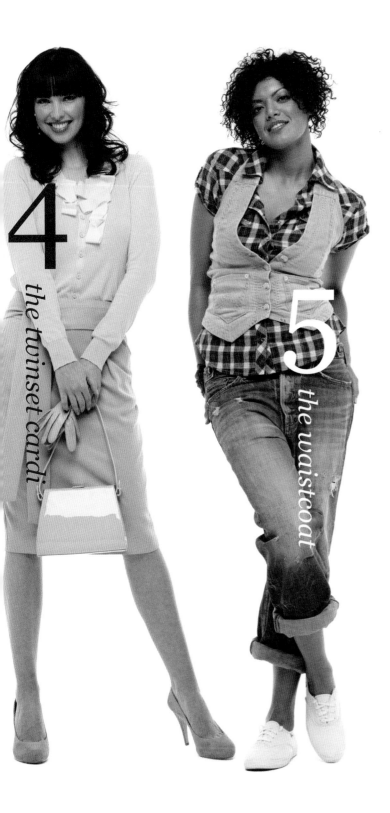

4 *the twinset cardi*

5 *the waistcoat*

> Use classic tops to totally alter the feel of your style – whether smart, casual or glam!

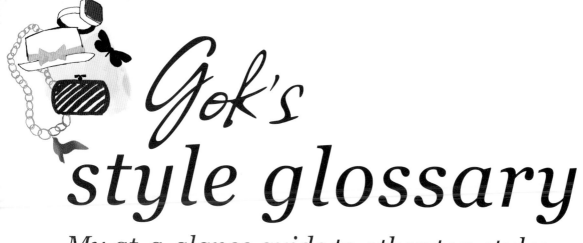

Gok's style glossary

My at-a-glance guide to other top styles

THE POLONECK

- **THE LOOK:** chic beatnik or preppy New Yorker.

- **WEAR WITH:** black capri pants and ballet pumps for a look that never dates (just add your fave handbag and some platforms to bring it up to date), or a pencil skirt and killer stilettos for classic office chic.

- **GOOD FIT FOR:** petites – the capri-pant version of the look will suit your figure down to a T; the pencil skirt look is great for curvy and pear-shaped girls as it will highlight their shapely outline.

- **NOT THE BEST FIT FOR:** tummy-shy babes, who might find this look tricky as it can shorten the frame and draw attention to the middle area; those with long or short necks could also struggle as polonecks draw attention to the length of the neck.

- **FAMOUS FOR WORKING THE LOOK:** Angelina Jolie, Audrey Hepburn.

86

THE BLOUSE

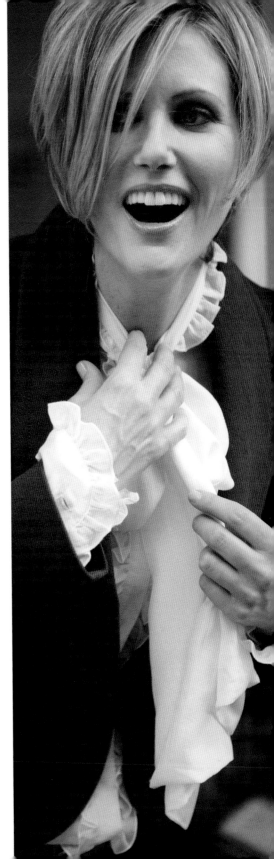

- **THE LOOK:** any gorgeously girlie top in a floaty or silky fabric, a pretty print or with delicate detail. The message? Ladylike chic, glam day-to-night.

- **WEAR WITH:** jeans for everyday elegance, or tailored suits, trousers and skirts for a chic workwear take. Add stilettos and a waistcoat if you want to look smarter.

- **GOOD FIT FOR:** petites who want to add volume on top (try a fitted blouse with big sleeves); bellissimo and bootylicious babes who want to cover their tums (wear a style that's neat at the shoulders but has flowing fabric that reaches below the stomach).

- **NOT THE BEST FIT FOR:** my lovely larger ladies – the silky fabrics will cling, not skim.

- **FAMOUS FOR WORKING THE LOOK:** Madonna, SJP and Dita von Teese.

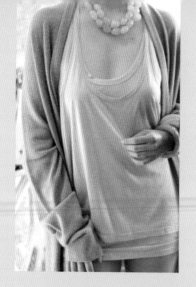

A little word about ...
LAYERING

WHEN I WAS ON THE JOB TRAINING TO BE A STYLIST, UNDERSTANDING HOW TO LAYER CLOTHES WAS ONE OF THE TRICKIER THINGS TO GET TO GRIPS WITH. But once I did, girls, I was amazed at how this styling device can double up the style factor. The basic idea is to wear tops of different lengths and shapes together. So you might buy a light, long vest that covers your bottom in one colour, then wear a shorter one in a different shade over it: the layering will instantly change the neckline and the bottom of your top and is a great way to cover up your not-so-good-bits while wearing shorter styles. Because layering always adds a modern touch, it's also a great way of bringing tired outfits up to date. There's no tried and tested rule, though — the best way to get a feel for layering is to experiment and figure out the combinations that work for you. That's what I do!

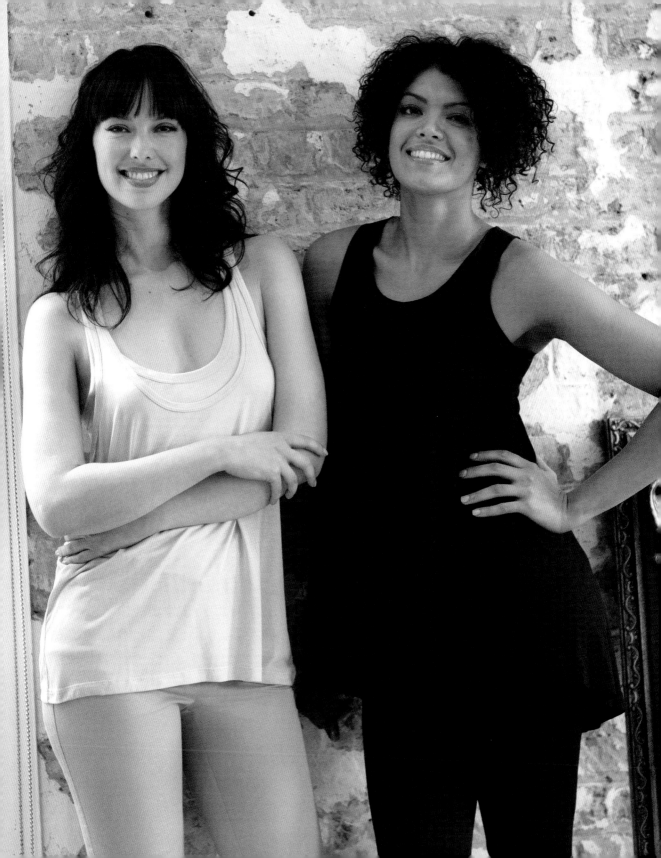

SAVVY SAVER

SPRUCE UP YOUR TOPS WITH MY TOP TIPS AND ADD A WHOLE NEW SHOT OF STYLE TO YOUR WARDROBE:

1 IF YOU HAVE A BIG, BAGGY T-SHIRT LURKING IN YOUR WARDROBE, PULL IT OUT AND ROLL UP THE SLEEVES. Fix them loosely with a big stitch and then cut the neck off the T-shirt to give it a soft, slouchy neckline. Loop a big, cotton scarf round your neck for a designer T-shirt take.

2 OLD WHITE COTTON TEES TAKE DYE REALLY WELL and since companies such as Dylon offer subtle colour palettes, it really is worth giving last year's tired-looking T-shirts a revitalising bolt of colour. Go for a really bright T-shirt and dress it up with bold accessories. Or, my girls who prefer to tone it down in the day can stick to classic tones, such as navy or grey.

3 WHETHER YOU WANT TO ADD A FOLKY, BOHO FEEL OR A HINT OF GLITZY GLAM, twinset cardies can really be brought back to life by adding some pretty trimming around the neckline. And, my sassy savers, you don't have to be Seamstress of the Year to stitch these on.

SAVVY SHOPPER

IF YOU'RE LOOKING TO FRESHEN UP YOUR CURRENT COLLECTION OF TOPS, JUST FOLLOW MY TOP SHOPPING TIPS:

1 YOU CAN PICK UP SOME GREAT BARGAIN CASHMERE CARDIES IN VINTAGE STORES. Look out for jewel-bright colours, such as emerald green and raspberry. They are a sweet accompaniment to prom dresses and skirts.

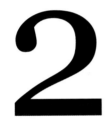

2 WHILE I THINK OUR GREAT BRITISH HIGH STREET CAN RIVAL MOST DESIGNER LOOKS, bargain acrylic knitwear can get tatty pretty quickly. If you want lots of wear out of your cardie, think about spending a little more, ladies. Look for 100 per cent wool, or cashmere-, silk- and cotton-mixes.

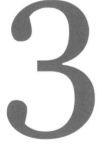

3 IF YOU'VE NEVER REALLY THOUGHT ABOUT WEARING A WAISTCOAT, go into your local department store and head for the designer rails. Designer collections often include waistcoats, but rather than just create straightforward suiting styles, these will have interesting details or will be cut in a different way. It's a great way to get some fab ideas for new ways to wear yours, my angels.

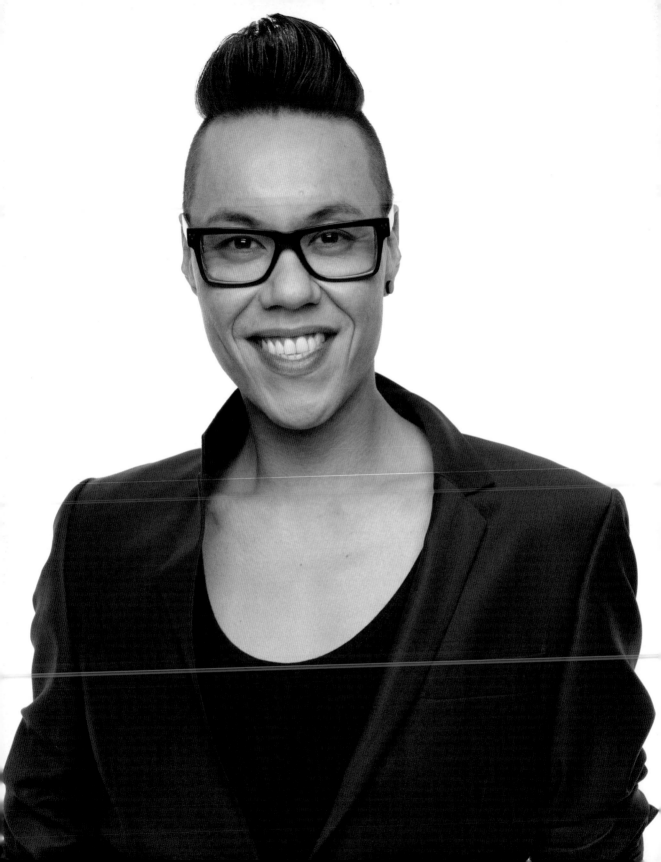

where to buy

FIND T-SHIRTS AT: Topshop, John Lewis, Joseph, Diesel, Oasis, Reiss   **FIND CARDIGANS AT:** Uniqlo, ASOS, Littlewoods Direct, Jaeger   All Saints   **FIND WAISTCOATS AT:** ASOS, Next, Vivienne Westwood Anglomania, Karen Millen, Lee, Wrangler   **FIND BLOUSES AT:** Gap, Levis, Jaeger, Whistles, Dorothy Perkins, Oasis, Miss Sixty, Zara   **FIND POLONECKS AT:** Joseph, Oasis, John Lewis, House of Fraser

"

From spring and summer to autumn and winter trends, we will look at some more fabulous ways to style up your tops in my *Timeless Style* section on page 194.

"

dresses
&
skirts

THEY'RE FAB, FEMININE AND GORGEOUSLY GLAM – of all the garments hanging up in your wardrobe, girls, there's nothing like a fave dress or skirt to make you feel oh-so-feminine. Designers have put them in the spotlight over the past few years, and the good news for you, my lovelies, is that the high street has followed suit.

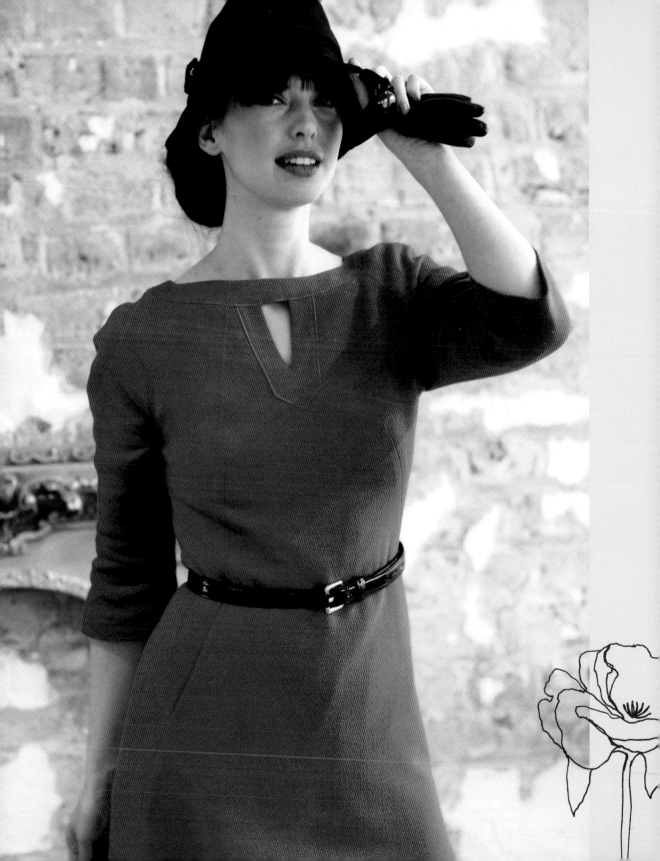

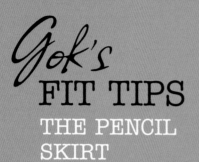

Gok's FIT TIPS

THE PENCIL SKIRT

1. A perfectly fitted pencil skirt hugs the body in all the right places and will look gorgeous – if it's too tight, though, your skirt will cling in all the wrong ones.

2. If you're petite or have chunky calves, choose a skirt that sexily skims the knee; longer pencil skirts – such as ones that skim the calf – can make you look shorter.

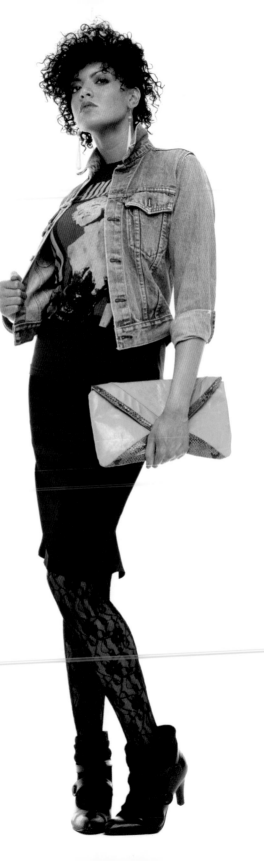

96

FROM RED-CARPET DAZZLERS TO THE DREAM SUMMER SHIFT, DRESSES ARE THE SELF-CONTAINED FASHION FIX OF ANY WARDROBE: a one-stop route to looking good. Skirts also throw up a trunk full of fashion options (which is perfect for all you ladies with a trunk full of them in your wardrobes!). From floor-skimming to thigh-slimming, I'll bet you have loads of top dresses and skirts that you've not worn for ages. So, whether you are in your trendy teens or your sexy sixties, let's work those styles and make them rock around the clock for you.

HERE ARE FOUR GREAT STYLES, AND EIGHT GREAT WAYS TO WEAR THEM:

1 *the pencil skirt*

NOW, LADIES, IF YOU DON'T ALREADY OWN A PENCIL SKIRT, THEN I'D SERIOUSLY SUGGEST THAT YOU GET ONE. This is the sexiest skirt shape on the planet and it's going to make you look pretty damn sexy, too, gorgeous. Whether you are a juicy pear shape, a curvy angel or a pretty petite, your pencil skirt will hug your curves and come in at the waist, creating a heavenly hourglass shape as it skims your body. And because pencil skirts have got serious classic credentials, they are great for chic day looks, elegant evenings and office-to-party dos.

• NOT SO PRIM AND PROPER
Because of its nice, neat shape, the pencil skirt is just crying out to have the primness shaken out of it, and I'd do this by adding some casual elements and

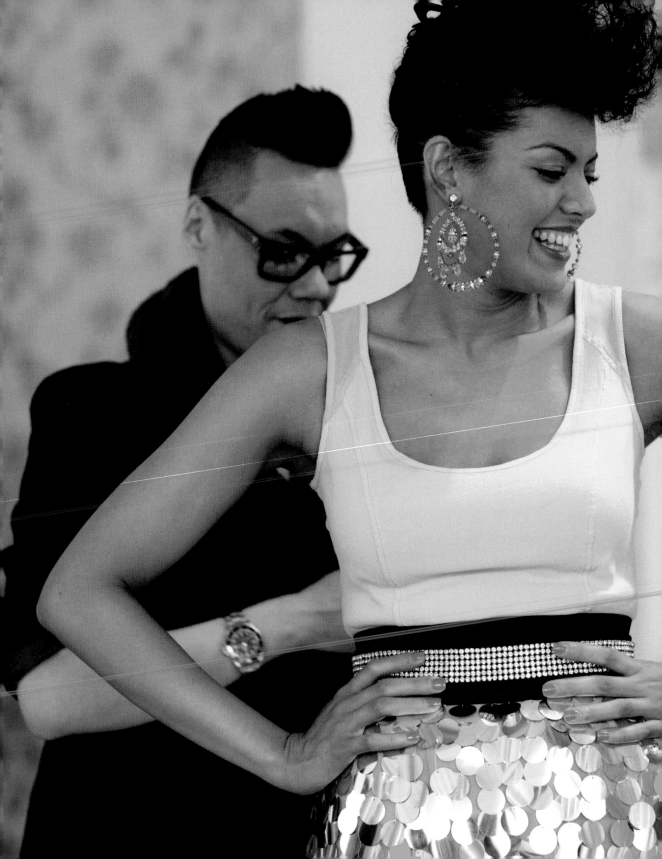

"Clasp on a big jewel-encrusted belt around the waist."

tougher textures. So, instead of going down the super-sexy route, think about wearing a T-shirt or your white shirt on top and then sling a leather biker jacket on. This is a great get-up for school-run mums: even the headmistress would approve! Or for a simpler take, wear a knitted top with your skirt and a pair of ballet flats. A stripy top will look the epitome of Parisian chic, too.

• SWEET AND SULTRY

This is a sensational look for a night out. Wear an off-the-shoulder top or a peasant-style blouse with puffy sleeves, and clasp a big statement jewel-encrusted belt high up on the waist. (A high-waisted pencil skirt will clinch the look, too.) Just add a fab pair of peep-toe heels. Or wear your pencil skirt with a sparkly top. And you can always keep your outfit all black for a demure approach (go for a black sequined top for evenings). For summer-evening glam, pin a foxy flower to your hair, or stitch one to a piece of sumptuous satin ribbon and tie around your neck, sultry señorita.

1. A prom skirt skims the hips and so is a great glam option for all my perfect pears.

2. Wide skirts flatten a big booty and balance out curvy cleavages, too. Heels will heighten the slimming power, girls.

3. Because all that volume speaks volumes, keep everything else you wear with a wide skirt as simple as possible.

2 *the wide skirt*

MANY OF MY GIRLS TELL ME THAT THEY LOVE WEARING SKIRTS WITH A LITTLE MORE VOLUME BECAUSE THEY HAVE SUCH A LADYLIKE FEEL. I get where you are coming from, girlfriends: there is something so fabulously flirty about swishy skirts. Even better, whether you go for a sophisticated A-line or a big and bouncy prom style, there are loads of ways to wear wider skirt shapes. There are so many options to choose from with this style – from dirndl to pleated and straight, so it's important to find the right fit for your figure. (See my 'Fit Tips' for pointers.) As the looks are endless, here are a couple to set you on your stylish way.

• EASY DOES IT
Wide skirts are great for getting that classic Grace Kelly look – add a fine-knit sweater, a pearl necklace and some mid-height heels or ballet flats. But although it looks lovely in pictures, you need

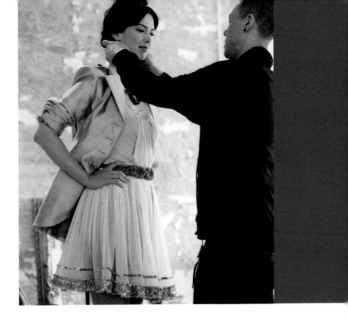

> *Whether you go for A-line or prom style, there are loads of ways to wear a wider skirt.*

to add some modern touches to make this look work now. Go for a skirt that has a bold print – coloured stripes, for instance (or if you have a black skirt, opt for a bold-print top instead). Add drama with some giant hoop earrings and a pair of killer platforms. Or, if you're still hooked on classics, slip on a belt with a fabulous buckle and throw an oversized cardie over your shoulders. Just add gold ballet flats or wedges for SJP style.

• PROM PERFECT

I just love a prom skirt: all these bouncy layers are enough to bring out the beautiful ballerina in anyone. You can go to town with a prom-style. (You can never have too many layers as far as I am concerned!) Layer up with net underskirts to add as much volume as you want. In the evening, go a bit sexier by pairing your skirt with a figure-skimming top. And, if you are one of my gorgeous older girls, a softer A-line skirt with a simple V-neck top (push the sleeves up to the elbows), a pair of smart court shoes and piles of necklaces is a classic look for a lunch date.

101

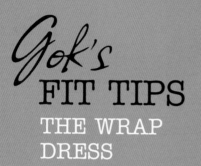

1. My apple-shaped girls, if you want to look seriously sexy in a wrap, get out your sculpting underwear to really cinch in that waist.

2. Wraps that have a belt that threads through the skirt will hold their shape more than those that just have ties at the front.

3. Cleavage divas look great in wraps as they make their boobs look fantastic, and the deep V, where the dress crosses over, adds sexiness. Perfect for girls who want to add curves up top.

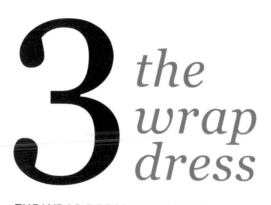

3 *the wrap dress*

THE WRAP DRESS HAS BECOME A REAL WARDROBE STAPLE FOR MOST OF MY GIRLS AND THAT'S PROBABLY BECAUSE IT'S SUCH A VERSATILE PIECE: you just slip it on, wrap it up and go. There is no better dress for covering any lumps and bumps because it really sculpts your body shape. The real beauty of this basic, though, ladies, is that not only is it a great daywear option, you can so easily smarten it up for lunch and dinner dates. What's more, if you have a black one in your wardrobe, you can whip up a wonderful party look in seconds — it's a brilliant backdrop for big, glitzy accessories.

• NICE AND SIMPLE

Printed wrap dresses are the easiest in the world to wear: bold patterns are such a statement that they do all the styling for you. So, for day, why not just keep things really simple by slipping on your wrap dress with a pair of knee-high boots. (Flats or heels work with wrap dresses.) Add a great day handbag and a short jacket for a shopping trip. Or, if you're going to the office, just slip on some court shoes or high strappy sandals. Add some statement jewellery to highlight that super-sexy neckline!

• NIGHT MOVES

The brilliant thing about wearing a wrap to evening dos is that while it packs a sexy punch, the freedom of the fabric makes it a really comfortable option. This instantly takes away that 'I'd never usually wear this' feeling that some of my girls say they get when they have to dress for formal occasions. The designer **DIANE VON FURSTENBERG** was the one who really made the wrap sexy when she dressed people such as Bianca Jagger in her slinky printed dresses in the seventies. Today, you can shine on in a really fabulous animal print or a dramatic patterned wrap dress by adding some diamanté earrings and a sparkly clutch and heels for that sultry seventies-siren look.

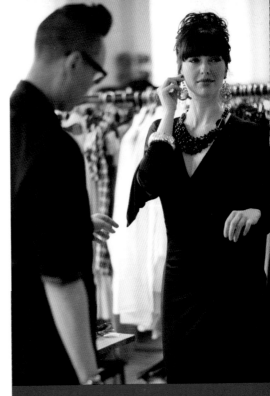

An evening-style wrap packs a sexy punch but is a comfortable option too.

103

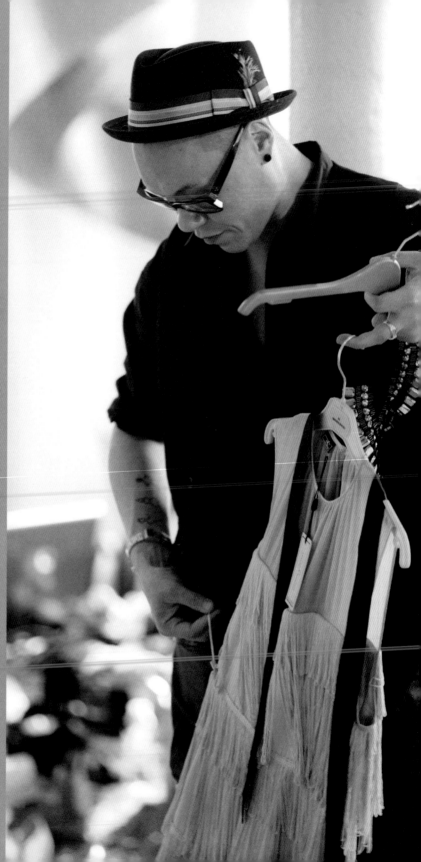

Gok's FIT TIPS

THE SHIFT DRESS

1. The perfect shift dress will fit neatly around your waist and taper to the knee, making the most of your lovely legs, gorgeous girls.

2. If it fits around your bust or stomach, it is likely to swing around your hips. Or if it fits around the hips, it may bag around your boobs. The bottom half of skirts and dresses are always easier to alter than the top, so, ladies, try to get the top-half fit right first.

4 *the shift dress*

IT IS ONE OF THE MOST RECOGNISABLE DRESS SHAPES IN FASHION HISTORY, and today the shift dress (which is basically cut in a straight-up-and-down shape and tapers down towards the legs) generally comes in two variations: a totally fitted sheath (like **AUDREY HEPBURN** in her famous LBD) or a slightly looser version, where it is not so fitted at the waist (great for covering tummies). Such a sensationally simple shape is easily interchangeable from day to night.

• SIXTIES CHICK

The shift is a brilliantly ageless look, ladies – pep up a plain shift by wearing a white shirt or a slinky poloneck underneath. Or pair it with a peplum jacket (one that nips in at the waist with a frilled hemline) for **JACKIE O**-style chic. A more funky retro take is to go for the looser style and wear a simple, shorter shift with opaque tights (a bold colour will look fab) and a pair of cute Mary Janes or boots.

• SEXY CHICK

Longer shifts that cling fabulously to your figure have got that lovely fifties feel to them. I would just add to that by heightening that hourglass shape with some sexy stockings. You can keep it that simple, or add a waist-cincher to bring your waist in further, or a fake-fur shrug for a real retro feel. Alternatively, keep legs bare (if you're pale, a touch of fake tan will work wonders) and slip on some glossy nude heels. Go for classic accessories, simple stilettos and a clutch bag.

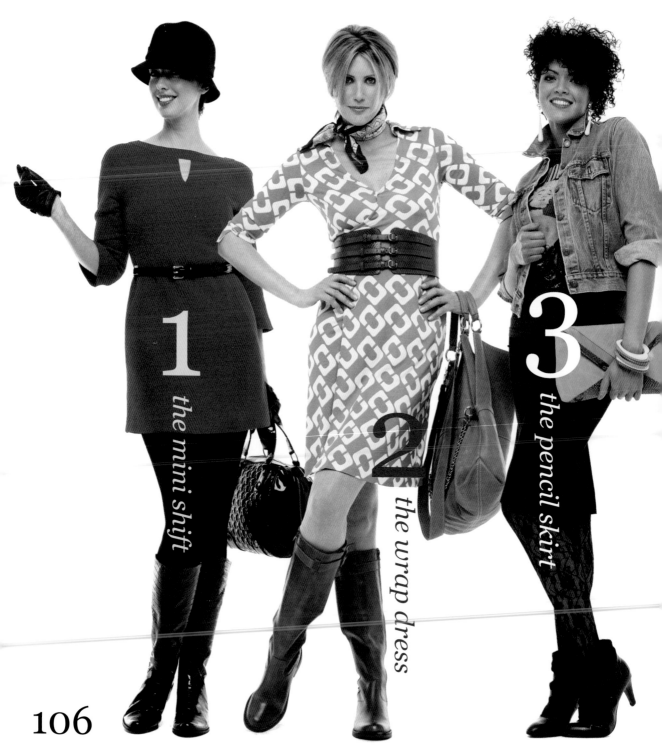

1 *the mini shift*

2 *the wrap dress*

3 *the pencil skirt*

106

WORK YOUR WARDROBE

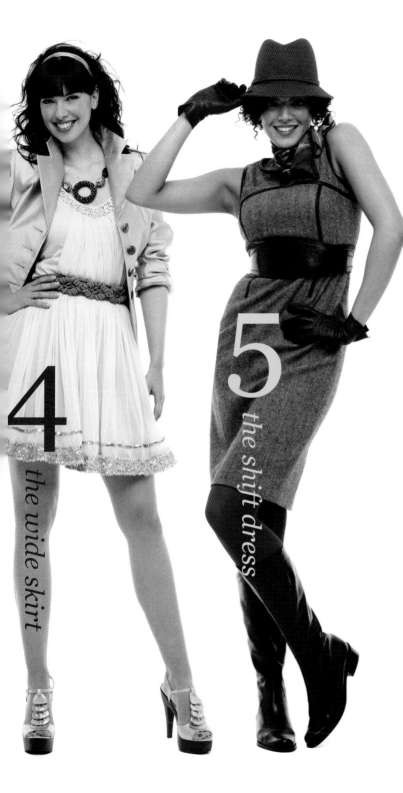

4

the wide skirt

5

the shift dress

"There's nothing like a gorgeous dress or skirt to make you feel simply gorgeous, too."

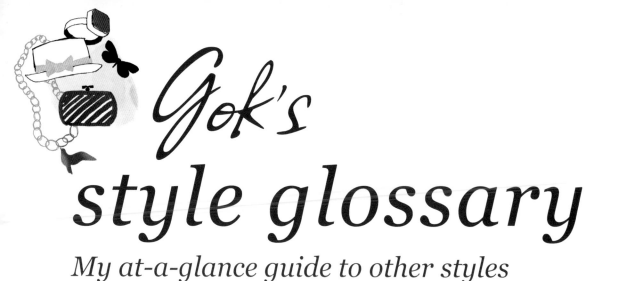

Gok's
style glossary

My at-a-glance guide to other styles

THE MAXI DRESS

- **THE LOOK:** full-length and fabulous.

- **WEAR WITH:** perfectly chosen accessories – gold Roman flats, or high jewelled sandals (but make sure the dress falls over them, so that your toes are showing when you walk).

- **GOOD FIT FOR:** all my girls who want to streamline their look in a show-stopping way. Maxis where the fabric flows from the bust are great for curvy or pear-shaped babes; figure-skimming styles are best for boyish, petite and slim fashionistas.

- **NOT THE BEST FIT FOR:** my sexy tall girls – it could stretch you an inch too far.

- **FAMOUS FOR WORKING THE LOOK:** J-Lo, Beyoncé and Elizabeth Hurley.

WORK YOUR WARDROBE

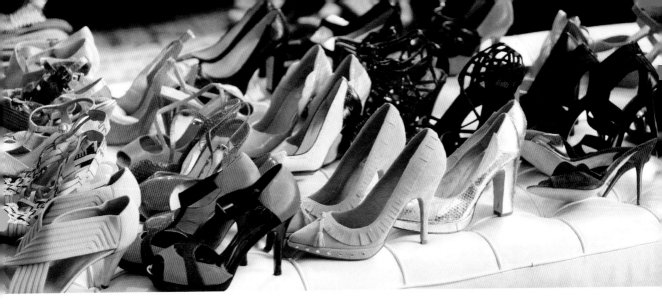

THE SHIRT DRESS

- **THE LOOK:** This dress, which is tailored but casual, has a real uptown-girl feel. It's a sassy and smart option for lunch dates.

- **WEAR WITH:** ballet pumps or thong sandals for a casual day look, or high-heeled pumps or wedges for a smarter take. A fabulous handbag and sunglasses will add sophistication.

- **GOOD FIT FOR:** my tummy-shy and straight-up-and-down girls: you can belt a shirtdress at the slimmest part of your waist, or on the hip to hide a wobbly tum. It's a sweet look for petites, too. Roll up the shirtsleeves to draw attention to the waistline.

- **NOT THE BEST FIT FOR:** cleavage divas – the buttons could gape at the bust – or booty babes – the neat top fit could throw your bottom half out of proportion.

- **FAMOUS FOR WORKING THE LOOK:** Kate Moss, Kirsten Dunst.

109

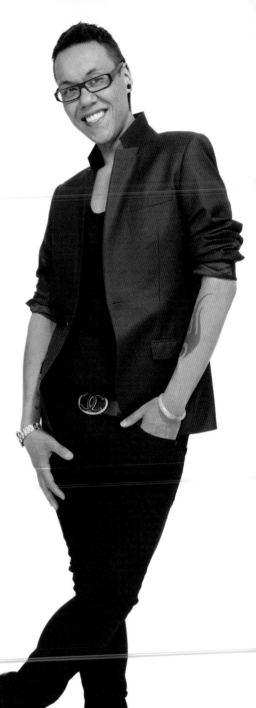

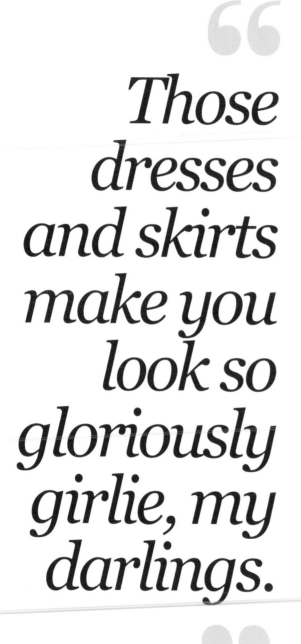

> *Those dresses and skirts make you look so gloriously girlie, my darlings.*

110

THE MINI SHIFT

- **THE LOOK:** short and sweet.

- **WEAR WITH:** gorgeously glossy bare pins or opaque tights. High-waisted bell-shaped minis look great with close-fitting tops; body-skimming sporty minis will work with a tight or a voluminous top.

- **GOOD FIT FOR:** anyone with shapely or long pins, and for trendy teens.

- **NOT THE BEST FIT FOR:** pear-shaped beauties or bootylicious girls – the mini proportions will have an unbalancing maxi effect.

- **FAMOUS FOR WORKING THE LOOK:** Kate Moss, Gwyneth Paltrow and Girls Aloud.

where to buy

FIND PENCIL SKIRTS AT: Reiss, River Island, ASOS, My-wardrobe.com

FIND WIDE SKIRTS AT: French Connection, Malene Birger, Next

FIND WRAP DRESSES AT: Diane Von Furstenberg, Issa, M&S **FIND SHIFT DRESSES AT:** M&S, Littlewoods Direct, Oasis, Karen Millen **FIND MAXI DRESSES AT:** Monsoon, ASOS, Debenhams, Topshop **FIND SHIRT DRESSES AT:** ASOS, Miss Selfridge, M&S **FIND MINI SHIFTS AT:** Topshop, H&M, ASOS

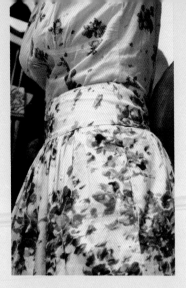

A little word about ...
PRINTS

FROM PAINTERLY SPLASHES TO PRETTY POLKA DOTS AND SASSY STRIPES,
printed skirts and dresses create instant style. There's no doubt that a great print will really get you noticed, whether you are walking the red carpet or walking to the shops. And, my lovelies, if you do a little print prep, you'll soon recognise the patterns that will pack a pretty punch for you. So, while a small, pretty, spriggy floral print will add an air of forties chic to my straight-up-and-down beauties, really curvy girls might find that they need a bolder print to stop them looking frumpy. (Smaller prints can fill out curvy shapes and have an ageing effect, while bigger, bolder ones balance proportions and have a more modern touch.) Pretty petites can also carry off bigger, bolder patterns, such as giant florals. My juicy pears might prefer to go for a skirt with a bold print and pair it with a plain top – the print will flatter your bottom half, while the simple top will create a clean, shapely line.

112

"A pretty print will really get you noticed."

SAVVY SAVER

IF ALL YOUR SKIRTS AND DRESSES NEED IS A LITTLE DRESSING UP, HERE ARE SOME WAYS TO DO IT:

1 YOU CAN REALLY CHANGE THE LOOK OF A DRESS THAT'S A FEW YEARS OLD BY ALTERING THE HEM. If it has a wide skirt, hem it to just above the knee – now you've got a classic summer dress.

2 REVITALISE YOUR WRAPS AND SHIRTDRESSES IN ONE SINGLE STEP: wear a different belt to the one that comes with the dress. A vintage silk scarf also looks good used as a belt on plainer styles.

3 CREATE SHOULDER STRAPS ON A SLEEVELESS OR PROM DRESS BY CUTTING SOME FABRIC OFF THE HEM, placing it round your neck (in halterneck style) and stitching it to the front of the bodice, then pinning a brooch at either side.

4 CHECK THE RAILS OF YOUR LOCAL CHARITY SHOP FOR SOME FABULOUS FITTED FIFTIES-STYLE SKIRTS AND DRESSES IN GOOD-QUALITY FABRICS. You can often pick up some great sixties shifts, too. Have them altered to fit and they'll look good as new.

SAVVY SHOPPER

YOU'LL ALWAYS FIND CLASSIC DRESS AND SKIRT SHAPES ON THE HIGH STREET. HERE ARE SOME OF THE DETAILS TO LOOK FOR:

1 A GREAT SHIFT WILL FIT YOUR SHAPE LIKE A GLOVE, though it's a tough call trying to find one. Buy the best fit you can and then get it altered so that it is tailored to fit your body.

2 WHEN BUYING SKIRTS, LOOK FOR ONES WITH LINING – they will hang better, feel nicer and won't cling to your legs.

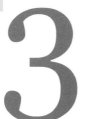

3 MOST HIGH-STREET STORES DESIGN A SATIN PENCIL SKIRT FOR THE PARTY SEASON but remember that satin is a really unforgiving fabric, so have a good think before you buy.

4 HAVE A GOOD IDEA OF WHERE YOU WILL WEAR YOUR SKIRT OR DRESS MOST so that you can picture what height heel or style of jacket it will work with.

5 SOME PRINTS ARE TIMELESS: florals, stripes and geometrics have classic appeal, while painterly splashes and neon brights could date quickly.

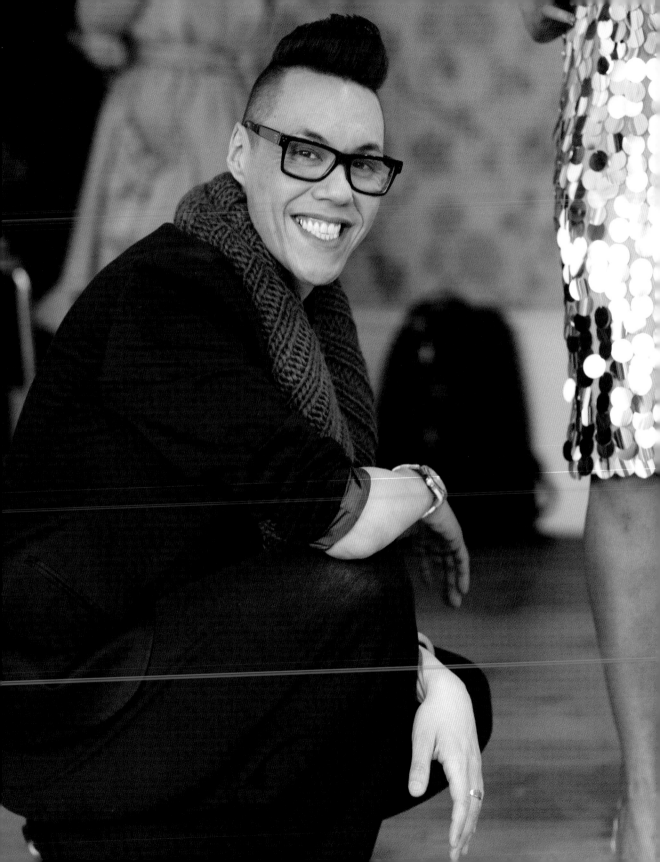

" I could fill this book with talk about dresses and skirts, ladies – there are so many styles to have fun with – but at least I have given you some great starting points for styling yours up. There are more delectable outfit options to come. So read on, my lovelies!

"

jackets & coats

TAKE IT FROM ME, GIRLS, whether it's a winter warmer, a short summer blazer or a cool, casual cover-up, jackets and coats are heroes of reinvention: and that means you don't have to spend, spend, spend to give the ones hanging in your wardrobe a fresh lease of life.

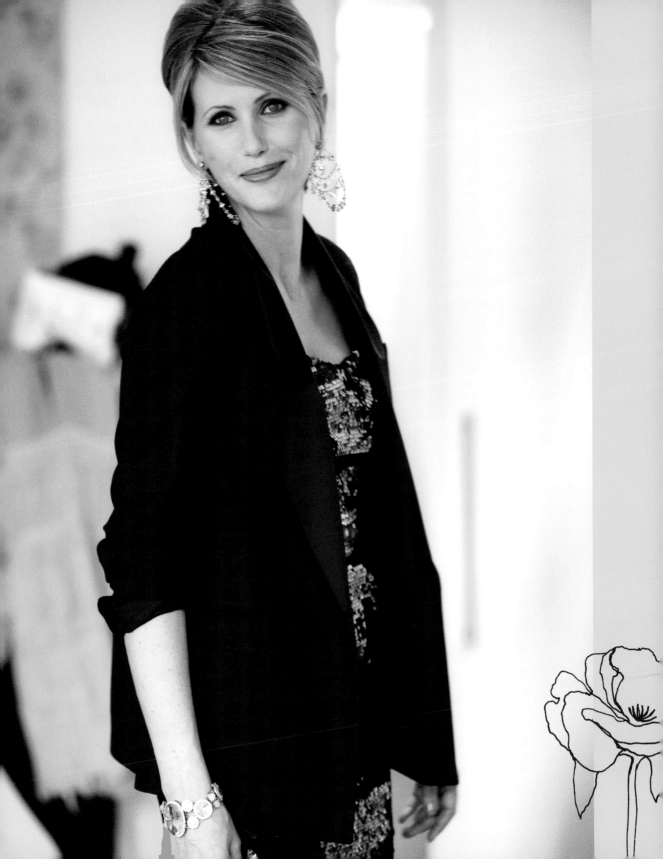

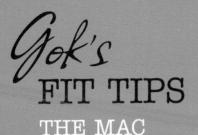

Gok's FIT TIPS

THE MAC

1. A mac that is too tight will spoil the look, ladies, so don't be afraid to go a little bigger in size with this style, as you need some fabric to gather in at the waist.

2. Macs that are hemmed just above the knee are great for most shapes, as they highlight legs at the sexiest spot. Just don your fave stilettos for a sexy touch.

3. If you're tummy is your trouble spot, belting your mac high above the waist will give a more nipped-in shape. Wear it loose and belted at the back for a casual take.

120

OF ALL OF THE GARMENTS HANGING IN YOUR CLOSET, YOU PROBABLY SHELL OUT MORE ON COATS AND JACKETS THAN ANY OTHER. And yet coats are the forgotten heroes of many wardrobes: not only do coats and jackets keep us warm, they add a fashionable flourish to any look. They are key to building up your style, girls, and yet I'm always surprised at how many of the lovely ladies I meet will spend ages putting together a fantastic outfit, only to undo all their elegant efforts by throwing on the nearest jacket that comes to hand at the end.

Let's take a look at **THREE CLASSIC STYLES** to work into your look.

1 *the mac*

OK, GIRLS, A MAC IS AS CRUCIAL A PART OF YOUR WARDROBE AS YOUR JEANS: you can wear it from day to night, from spring through to winter, this year, next year – to 2050 and beyond! In fact, such are the style credentials of this wardrobe wonder that it would be a serious contender for the Lifetime

Achievement Award at my Fashion Oscars. Covering up with a mac in any of the classic shades – black, stone or navy – will always add a suave touch to casual or smart outfits. And, as mac fans from **CATHERINE DENEUVE** to **KATE MOSS** have shown us over the years, this classic coat is a seriously sexy option, too.

• DAY TRIPPER

Whether you are going shopping in town or popping out for a bite to eat with the girls, this casual mac look – which the British designer **MARGARET HOWELL** does brilliantly – is a great daywear choice. Tuck one of your fitted white shirts into a pair of chinos (or any of your casual trousers in a neutral tone), dig out a natural leather belt and roll the trouser hems up to just above the ankles. Depending on how much running around you are likely to be doing (hitting the shops can be hard work!), go for flat shoes (loafers and brogues are so on-trend right now), or add height and lengthen pins with some wedge sandals. Put your mac on and tie the belt loosely at the back of the coat. Get out your biggest handbag and pull on some giant sunglasses. Girlfriend, you are good to go!

• STYLISH AND SEXY

For sizzling evening style, show some leg, ladies: wear a belted mac over your favourite pencil skirt, so that the focus falls on your legs and – for the full voluptuous vamp effect – high, high heels. It's the kind of sultry siren look that *SEX AND THE CITY'S* **SAMANTHA** pulls off so fabulously. The belted waist shows off curves, and you can up the va-va-voom factor by rolling up your coat sleeves to the elbows and pulling up the collar. You're hot to trot, hot stuff!

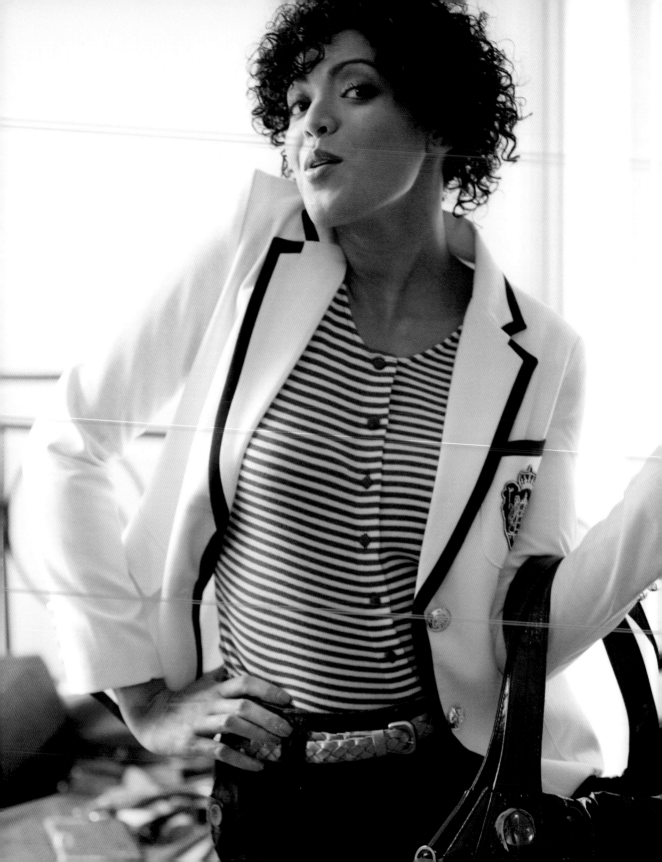

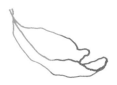

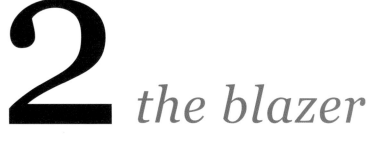

2 *the blazer*

IT'S MADE A BLAZING RETURN TO THE CATWALKS OVER THE PAST FEW SEASONS AND NOW THE CLASSIC TAILORED JACKET CAN BLAZE TO THE FRONT OF YOUR WARDROBE TOO, ANGELS. Whether it's in the form of a tux or a looser, oversized boyfriend blazer, this do-all cover-up will rise to any occasion. I always have one on standby when I am styling my girls, as not only can I pair it with jeans, skirts and dresses, I can take it from casual to glam in an instant. Here's how:

• SOFT TOUCH

Seamstresses hate me for it but sometimes I love tailored pieces to be a little on the baggy side, and that's the idea behind the modern blazer look, gorgeous girls: it shouldn't feel too structured. For day, just think soft layers, such as a baggy shirt or T-shirt, a casually looped scarf, loose-fitting jeans (give those boyfriends an outing) and plimsolls. Slip your blazer on top. Keep it straight on the bottom

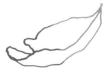

123

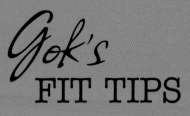

Gok's FIT TIPS

THE BLAZER

1. Single-breasted blazers are the most flattering for most shapes. Double-breasted styles are likely to do just that, my lovelies — double you in size.

2. Cropped blazers are better for petites and curvy girls: they won't swamp your frame, but they will highlight your gorgeous waist and elongate your legs.

3. If you like to show off your neck, or want to add fashionable flair, turn your collar up, sassy lady.

(a pencil skirt, shift dress or skinny trousers will work) for a sharp, tailored look. Or go for wide pants — but best whip out those heels and a good belt, ladies: they'll highlight your waist and stop you looking boxy on top.

• SMART CHOICE

Although blazers are generally thought of as daywear, they've become a real hit for evening events of late — I loved the way **GWYNETH PALTROW** dressed down a thigh-skimming mini dress and mega-heels with a long-length blazer at a red-carpet event. If you love to show off your pins, then you should go for that look, too, you brave babe! Or get the look with a show-stopping sequined blazer. If, however, you feel it's just not the style for you, then go the opposite way and wear your blazer with a floor-skimming dress instead. (This will only work with fishtail or bias-cut shapes, though, as you need the fabric to cling at the hip and sway out again so that your bottom half is well defined. Looser dress shapes will give you a SpongeBob SquarePants silhouette!) Throw your blazer on top, accessorise with your most gorgeous, glittery cocktail bag and some huge earrings, and shine on, glamour puss!

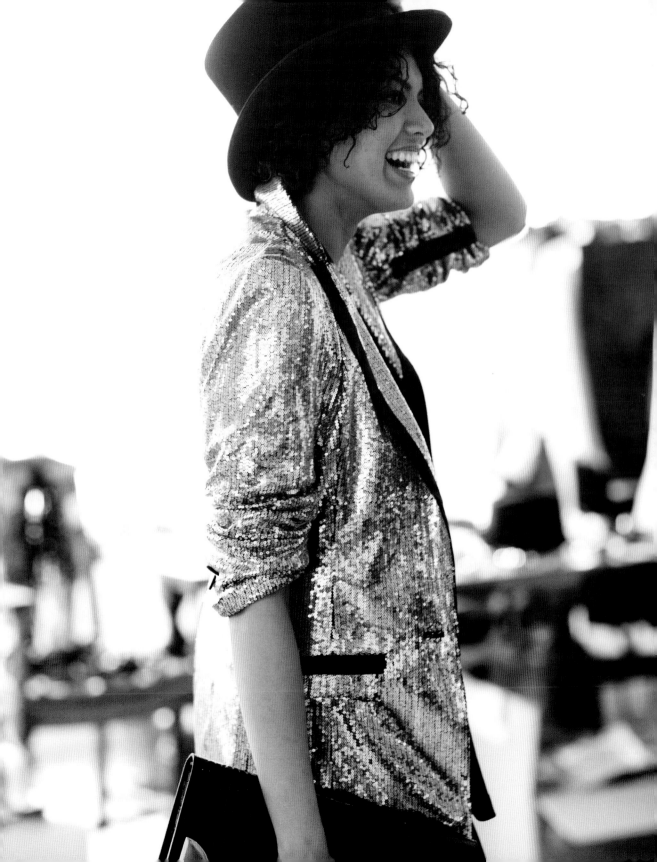

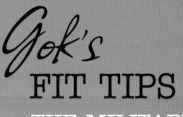

Gok's
FIT TIPS
THE MILITARY COAT

1. Frock coats look fab on you, my pretty pears: they will fit your shape well at the shoulders and waist, while skimming that troublesome thigh area.

2. Shorter pea-coat styles will look *très* chic on girls with great pins and anyone who wants to focus attention away from the stomach area – they add a little structure on top and will highlight your luscious legs.

3. In the warmer months, go for navy or white militaristic coats and jackets with gilt trim and buttons.

3 *the military coat*

FOR DAYS WHEN YOU WANT TO LOOK A LITTLE DRESSY BUT JUST DON'T HAVE THE TIME TO PUT ANY EXTRA WORK IN, BUSY BEAUTIES, A MILITARY-STYLE COAT WILL SMARTEN YOU UP PRONTO! It's the tailoring and detailing – ornate frogging, neat rows of brass buttons – that give these coats such an instantly groomed look. The benefit of these elegant embellishments, ladies? You can keep whatever you are wearing underneath as easy and simple as you like and let the coat do all the styling for you. And you don't have to join up to get kitted out, my military maidens, just adapt your existing coats and jackets to get the look.

• SUMMER PARADE
Traditionally, uniform-inspired styles always crop up on the catwalks in the winter months, but

recently braids, brass buttons and other militaristic details have been working their way into summer collections, too. If it's a look that makes you stand to attention, hot stuff, then a cropped cotton military blazer would be a great everyday jacket for those in-between-season days when there's a naughty nip in the air. With a jacket this smart, you can afford to go casual underneath: layer up with any of your long T-shirts (try a stripy one) and slip on your favourite jeans and flatties. Sling your slouchiest bag over your shoulder and march on!

• WINTER WARM

If you think the full-on military look is too strong for you, just add militaristic details with accessories. So pull all your old winter coats out of your wardrobe and look for one that comes in at the waist. (Tailoring is key here.) Add a touch of French Resistance chic with a gilt-detail belt and a little cap. Some patent ankle boots and a pair of fabulous gloves will add a dash of glossy glamour. For night, throw your coat over a long skirt or dress and slip on some high heels. (Make sure your dress covers them as if it's too short it will knock your shape off balance.) A red scarf will add fabulous forties-style flair.

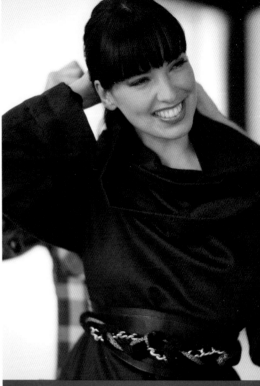

66

Tailoring and detailing give military coats an instantly groomed look.

99

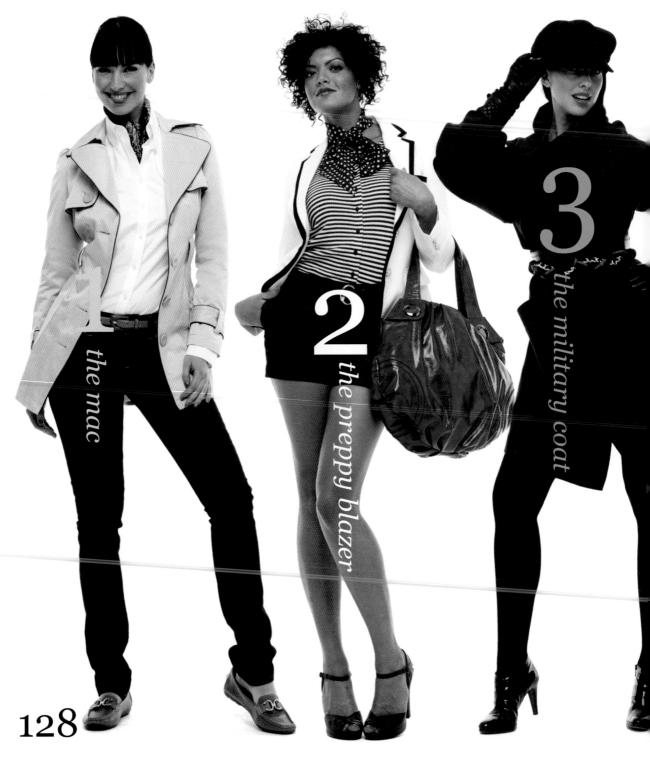

1 the mac

2 the preppy blazer

3 the military coat

WORK YOUR WARDROBE

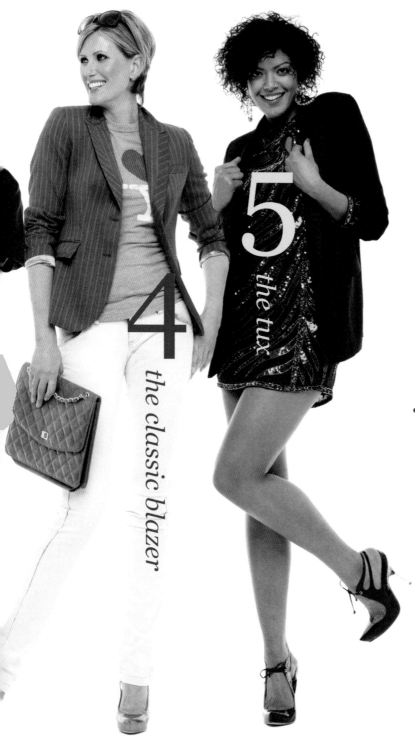

4 *the classic blazer*

5 *the tux*

> "You don't have to spend a fortune to give your coats and jackets a new lease of life."

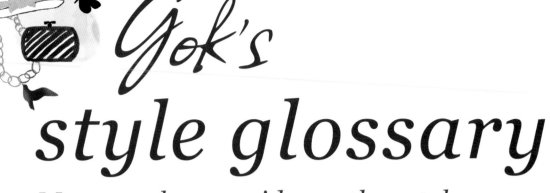

Gok's
style glossary

My at-a-glance guide to other styles

THE LEATHER JACKET

- **THE LOOK:** whether you're a smart chick or a rock chick, there's a leather jacket to suit your style.

- **WEAR WITH:** jeans and a white shirt; skinnies and a rock T-shirt; skirts and a vest for casual cool.

- **GOOD FIT FOR:** most shapes. Because leather jackets are not as structured as they used to be (you'll find softer, longer cuts and colours in high-street stores now), look around and find one that fits your figure.

- **NOT THE BEST FIT FOR:** my larger lovelies – you gorgeous girls should probably stay away from traditional biker styles as they can bring out a little too much of the biker bit. My older girls should stick to softer shapes and colours.

- **FAMOUS FOR WORKING THE LOOK:** Kate Moss, Alexa Chung.

THE STATEMENT COAT

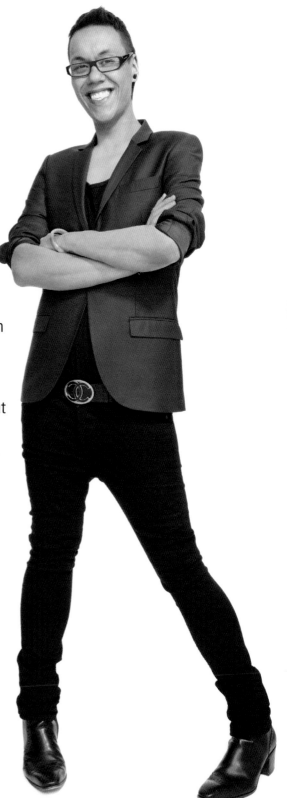

- **THE LOOK:** jewelled, patterned or brightly coloured – this elegant style is so ladylike in feel and shape, with lovely details such as three-quarter-length sleeves.

- **WEAR WITH:** plain skirts and tops in neutral or in bold colours, or an LBD in the evening.

- **GOOD FIT FOR:** curvy or big-busted girls, who should look for a straight cut that hangs from the shoulders; juicy pears, who will look great in a brightly coloured or metallic-sheen style that ties at the waist.

- **NOT THE BEST FIT FOR:** anyone who doesn't like the idea of 'look-at-me' style.

- **FAMOUS FOR WORKING THE LOOK:** Judi Dench, SJP and Michelle Obama.

SAVVY SAVER

RIGHT, GIRLS, IT'S TIME TO REACH INTO THAT WARDROBE AND GATHER THOSE OLD COATS AND JACKETS THAT YOU HAVE GIVEN UP ON. HERE ARE SOME EASY REINVENTION TIPS TO FRESHEN UP THOSE STYLES:

1 A TRADITIONAL BEIGE MAC IS A TIMELESS CLASSIC, but don't feel you have to treat it like a time capsule, gorgeous. Give it a great big boost of colour: dye it bright red.

2 IF YOU'VE GOT AN OLD WORK BLAZER THAT STOPS JUST BELOW YOUR BUM and simply looking at it makes you feel like frump of the year, have it shortened to just below your waist. You'll love its trendy new guise, girls.

3 I KNOW I'M ALWAYS SAYING IT, GIRLS, but changing the buttons can totally revamp a garment, and the blazer really lends itself to this mini makeover. Oversized buttons will add a trendy touch; brass or gilt ones will add 'in-the-navy' sass.

SAVVY SHOPPER

A COAT'S NOT JUST FOR CHRISTMAS, IT'S FOR LIFE! IT'S THE ITEM WE SPLASH MOST CASH ON, SO IF YOU ARE PLANNING TO SPLURGE, LADIES, HERE ARE A FEW THINGS TO BEAR IN MIND:

1 WHEN BUYING A COAT, DON'T FEEL YOU ALWAYS HAVE TO GO FOR BLACK TO MAKE IT LAST, LADIES – neutral tones, such as navy, stone and grey can really refresh your wardrobe and they have lasting power, too.

2 BLAZER STYLES SEEM TO CHANGE A LOT FROM SEASON TO SEASON, so, girls, work out whether you'll get more wear out of a short fitted one or a loose boyfriend style.

3 RATHER THAN SPLASH OUT ON A FULL-ON MILITARY-STYLE COAT WITH ALL THE DETAILS, invest in a long, neutral-coloured coat and adapt it when you want with belts and medal-style brooches, smart chick.

4 THE HIGH STREET HAS SOME GREAT-QUALITY WINTER COATS AT TOP-QUALITY PRICES. But while we all love a bargain, make sure that the coat you go for is well-made enough to keep you warm – though that Puffa won't cut it on the red carpet!

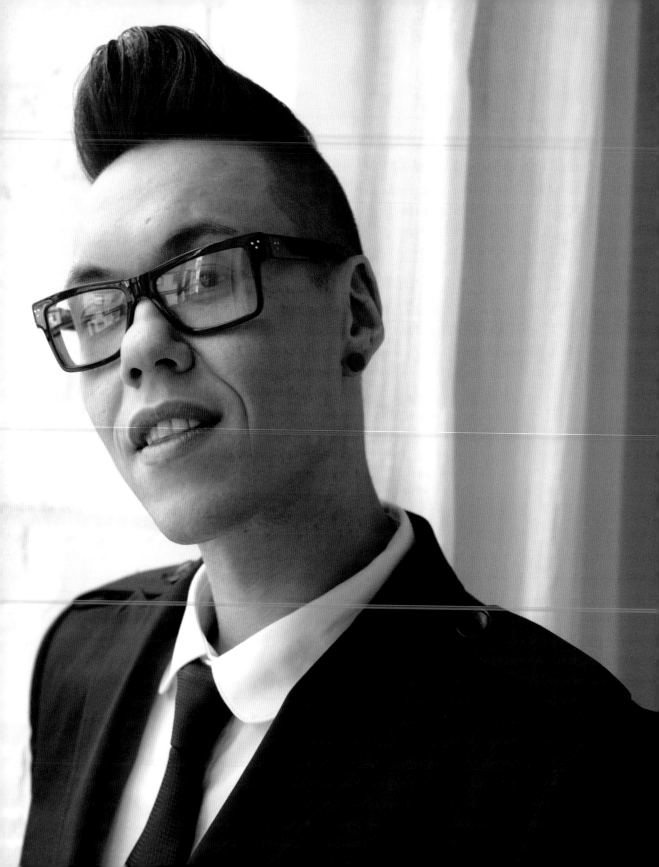

where to buy

FIND MACS AT: Gap, Debenhams, Topshop, Dorothy Perkins, Next, Zara, ASOS, APC   **FIND BLAZERS AT:** Topshop, Zara, River Island, Oasis

Uniqlo   **FIND MILITARY COATS AT:** Topshop, Karen Millen, Oasis, Jigsaw

FIND LEATHER JACKETS AT: Whistles, ASOS, All Saints, M&S

FIND STATEMENT COATS AT: Jaeger, Betty Jackson Black, M&S

"

Whatever look you are going for, my lovelies, when it comes to coats and jackets, we've got it all wrapped up.

"

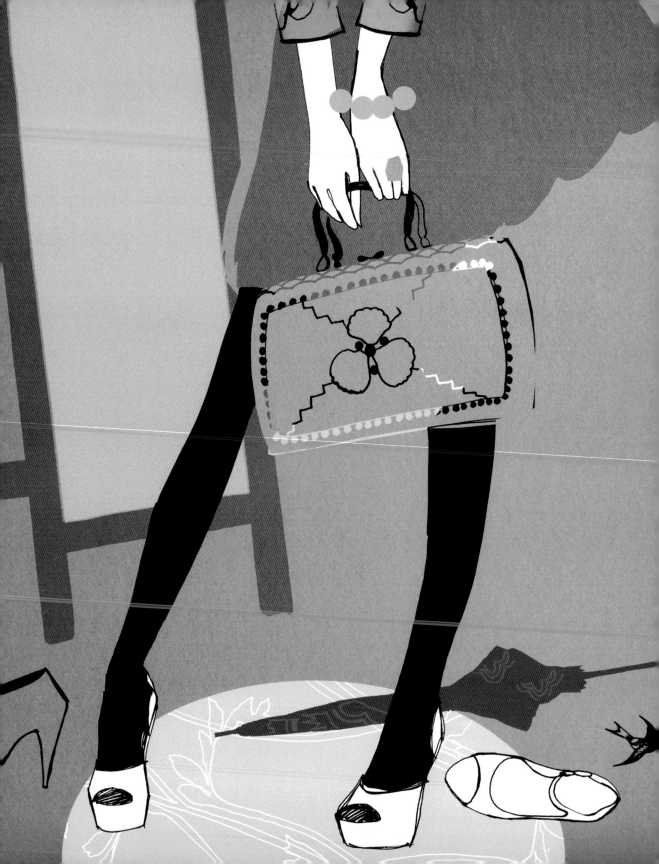

elegant
extras

From gorgeous handbags to heavenly heels and glittering jewels, let's add some fabulous finishing touches

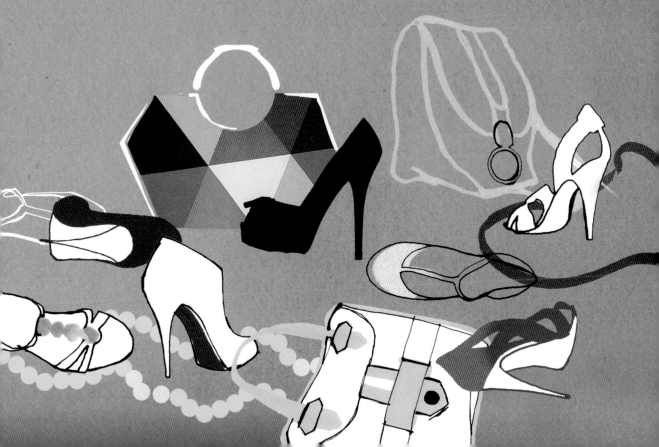

shoes & boots

OF ALL THE ACCESSORIES IN YOUR
WARDROBES, GIRLS, YOUR SHOES
REALLY DICTATE YOUR STYLE. So,
*whether it's a pair of red stilettos, gold
ballet pumps or those brilliant black boots
that you pull out every winter, let's style
them up to suit your look.*

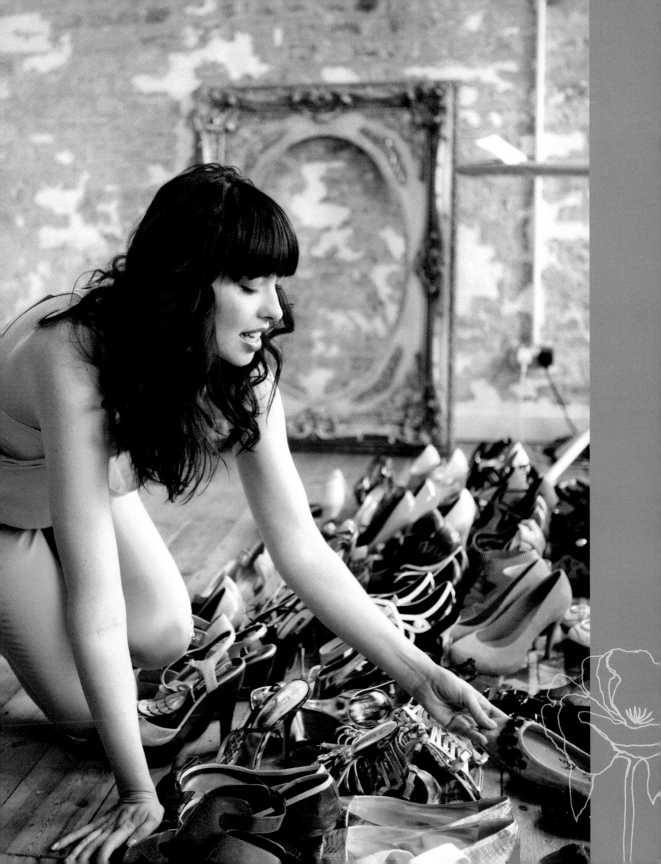

YOU DON'T HAVE TO BE A PARTICULAR AGE, SHAPE OR SIZE TO WEAR CERTAIN SHOE STYLES: shoes just have that all-round fabulous feel-good factor. If you have a fantastic pair of flats, a hot pair of heels and a brilliant pair of boots in that wardrobe, you will always be ready to step out in style.

Now, let's look at some of the classic **SHOE AND BOOT** styles. I'll also let you know where to buy them if you want to add some new pairs to your shoe line-up.

1. *flats*

• PLIMSOLLS

THE LOOK: Off-duty chic. OK, love 'em or loathe 'em, flat shoes are a necessity, because Sainsbury's in stilettos is a look that even Victoria Beckham might struggle to pull off. Flat, though, needn't mean frumpy. If you are a real jeans-and-jacket girl, plimsolls are a fashionable alternative to trainers. Keep those sporty styles for the gym, ladies!

WEAR WITH: jeans, floral summer dresses and denim skirts for off-duty chic.

STYLE NO-NO: if you are short or have wide calves, I'd say plimsolls are not the most flattering flats for you – open sandals and ballet flats show more skin and are a better choice.

FIND PLIMSOLLS AT: Converse, Superga, Keds.

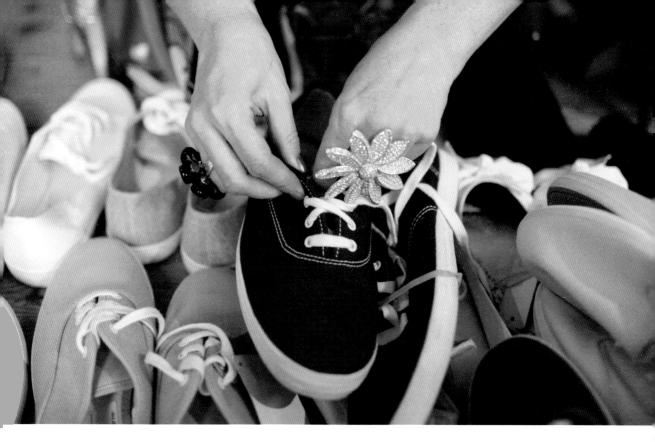

• LOAFERS

THE LOOK: Casual chic. You get loads of wear out of a good pair of loafers, and if you have some in tan or black leather, they will go well with trouser styles such as coloured or denim jeans or stone-coloured chinos.

WEAR WITH: boyfriend and straight jeans or chinos.

STYLE NO-NO: loafers are not great with skirts and dresses. Also, they can look a little masculine and widen calves, so make sure you feminise your look. Stick to ballet flats if you don't want to shorten legs.

FIND LOAFERS AT: Chloé, Blowfish, Office, Kurt Geiger, Patrick Cox.

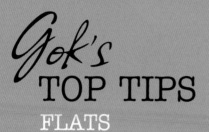

Gok's
TOP TIPS
FLATS

1. When wearing flats, watch your deportment – that oh-so-comfortable feeling can cause you to slouch.

2. Go for quilted, patent or buckle-front flats for a more uptown feel.

3. Elasticated or fold-up ballet flats look good and are a great help when you are wearing heels: you can wear them to walk to your destination, then slip heels on when you get there.

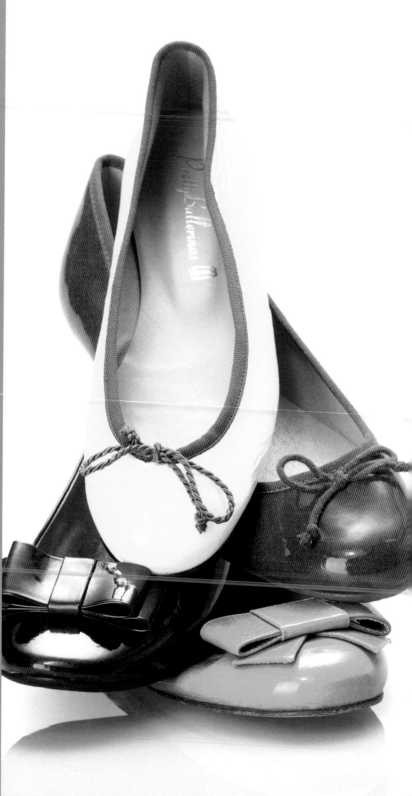

142

• BALLET PUMPS

THE LOOK: Everyday elegance. Since designers such as **MARC JACOBS** and **TORY BURCH** started adding funky little finishes to ballet pumps, they have become a staple in every fashionista's wardrobe. You can go as plain or as pretty as you like – these slip-on-and-go sensations will work with most outfits, and brightly jewelled, coloured or textured ones will take you from day to night with ease.

WEAR WITH: skinny and bootcut jeans, floral dresses, pencil skirts, capri pants and wide-leg trousers.

STYLE NO-NO: not great with maxi dresses.

FIND BALLET PUMPS AT: Juicy Couture, L. K. Bennett, Marc by Marc Jacobs, Pretty Ballerina, French Sole.

• SUMMER SANDALS

THE LOOK: Hot, hot, hot. We've come a long way from the flip-flop and jelly shoes that so often used to be your lot in a warm-weather sandal. Gladiator and thong styles are the most versatile style to own now. Go for those with jewels, stones and coloured detail for day-to-night appeal.

WEAR WITH: jeans, skirts, long dresses, short dresses and anything else you care to pair them with. Open sandals, such as slim thong styles that show lots of skin, are good for lengthening legs.

STYLE NO-NO: they won't work with smart or tailored styles.

FIND SUMMER SANDALS AT: Topshop, Office, Russell & Bromley, Gap, Faith.

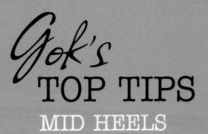

1. If you have wide calves, wedges or square heels would be a better choice for you than kitten heels, as they can really shorten the leg.

2. Peep toes are one of the most flattering mid-heel styles; the little shape at the front creates a flattering, lengthening line.

3. Mid-heel loafer styles with brass buckles are a chic alternative to plain black square heels for the office — and they'll work with jeans at the weekend.

2.mid heels

• COURT SHOES

THE LOOK: Everyday glam. You've probably got loads of mid-heel courts in your wardrobe that you've not worn for ages. If you're feeling a little ruthless, put these in the Oxfam pile, particularly anything with a square toe and square heel (it's not hip to be square!) and old-style low kitten heels (which can make your calves look squat. New ones are a little higher). What to keep? Any eighties-style cone heels (great with skinnies), high-ish stack heels (they'll work with that pencil skirt) and open-toe slingbacks (they always cut an elegant line). Try not to stick to black styles — experiment with nude tones or go for brights.

WEAR WITH: skinny jeans and trousers.

STYLE NO-NO: they don't work with wide-leg trousers — mid-heels can have a shortening effect on all but the tallest figures.

FIND MID-HEELS AT: Shelly's at ASOS, Office, L. K. Bennett, Marc by Marc Jacobs.

• WEDGES

THE LOOK: Contemporary chic. I have never, ever met a woman who doesn't appear more confident when wearing a block heel, and I've converted many a non-heel wearer to the wonder of the wedge! For a start, ladies, they give you longer-looking pins. They are also easier to walk in than heels. If you don't have some in your wardrobe already, then head for the high street. From easy espadrilles to catwalk-cruise chic and strappy block-heel sandals and pumps, there are just so many great options out there now.

WEAR WITH: block heels will work with most of your capsule wardrobe.

STYLE NO-NO: they won't do the business with black work trousers.

FIND WEDGES AND PLATFORMS AT: Gap, Office, Kurt Geiger, Topshop, French Connection.

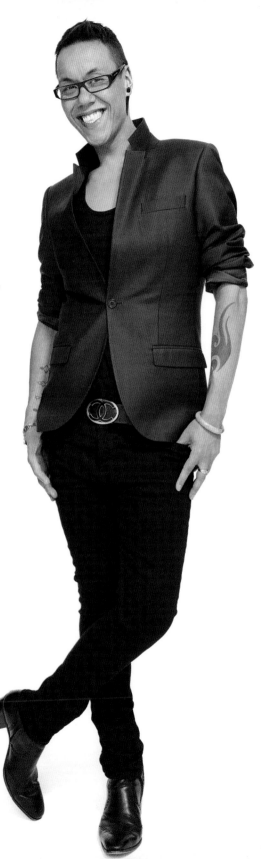

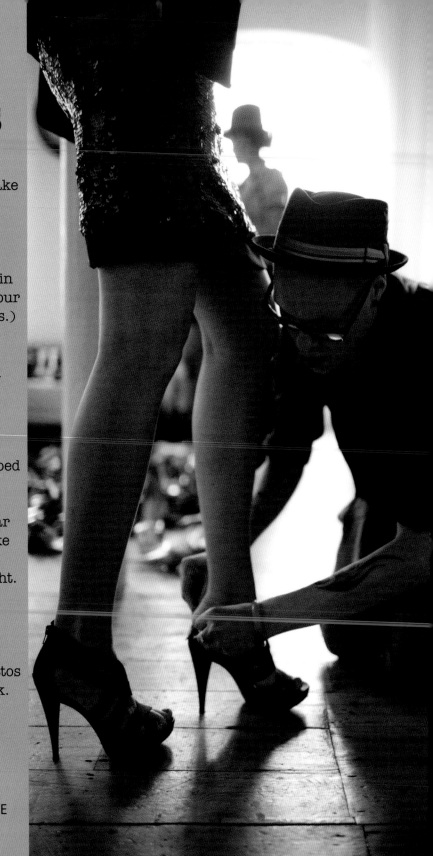

Gok's
TOP TIPS
HIGH HEELS

1. Heels instantly make you stand straighter, look taller and give your body a better shape. (For the full slimming effect, pull in your tum and hold your shoulders back, ladies.)

2. What heel size to wear? If you feel you are about to fall off, then your heels are too high. If you can't walk, you ain't going anywhere, my stilettoed sensation.

3. If you want to wear high, high heels, make sure you have a taxi on call the whole night.

4. Get stilettos re-heeled regularly to keep them looking smart – scuffed stilettos are never a good look.

146

3. *high heels*

• STILETTOS AND PLATFORMS

THE LOOK: Super-sexy. Now, I think every woman should have a pair of stilettos in her wardrobe, because this, the sexiest shoe of all, will make you feel that way, too. Not only do stilettos give legs and bum a boost, gorgeous, they make you feel instantly elevated – physically and mentally. In fact, classic stilettos are such an essential that I think every girl should get a pair free on the NHS! They don't have to be black – nude-toned patent stilettos look seriously sexy and are not as heavy as black, so are great for wearing with lighter colours. Or think about adding a bright pair to your wardrobe: shocking-pink, scarlet and electric-blue stilettos will add a super-sexy splash of colour to top-to-toe black. And if you find that teetering around in spiky stilettos is a balancing act too far, super-high, strappy platform styles are a great alternative as the block heel makes them far easier to walk in.

WEAR WITH: pencil and wide-hem skirts, skinny jeans and slim trousers.

STYLE NO-NO: stilettos can be tricky to pair with wide-leg trousers.

FIND STILETTOS AND PLATFORMS AT: Topshop, Next, Oasis, Karen Millen, Kurt Geiger, Dune, ALDO.

4.boots

• CLASSIC BIKER

THE LOOK: Comfortably cool. I just love classic biker boots, but if you wear them with full-on leathers, you'll look like you got lost on the way to your Harley-Davidson. The trick to making these cool classics work is to soften the look by pairing them with a floral dress and opaque tights, or wearing a pretty blouse and jeans.

WEAR WITH: jeans and dresses (shorter boot styles) or wide-hem and pencil skirts (longer boot styles). Shorter styles can shorten legs, so remember to choose carefully to suit your shape.

STYLE NO-NO: don't wear with leather trousers or smart outfits.

FIND BIKER BOOTS AT: Carvela, R. Soles, Office, ASOS, ALDO, Bertie.

• RIDING BOOTS

THE LOOK: Whip smart. Classic riding-boot styles are probably more expensive than any other, so, my angels, if you have a pair of these tucked away for winter, chances are that you splashed a bit of cash on them. Investment buys like this are worth every penny: riding-boot styles hold their shape well and are designed to fit the curve of the leg, giving your pins a great silhouette. Plus, that high-polished leather always adds a luxurious touch.

"

Investment
buys like
riding boots
are worth
every penny!
They give
your pins a
fab silhouette.

"

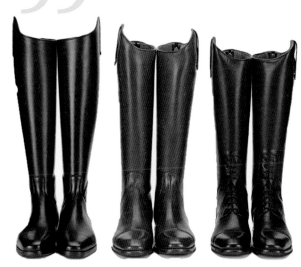
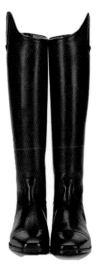

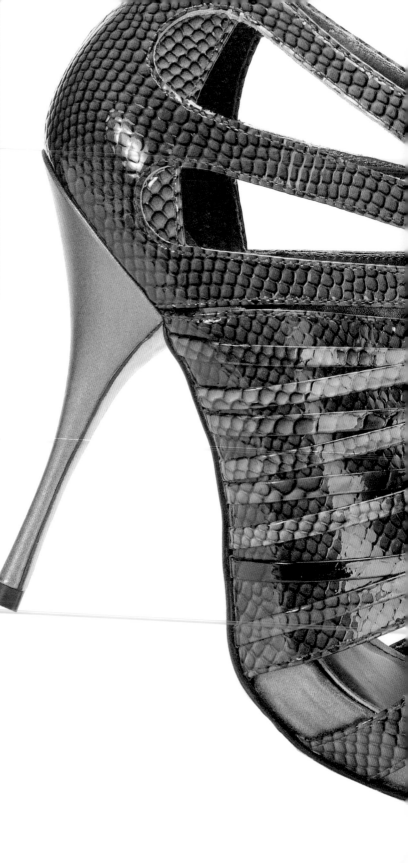

Gok's TOP TIPS

BOOTS

1. If you have trouble getting boots to fit round your calves, there are many specialists offering larger styles or personal fitting services. Here are just a few: **Duoboots.com, Emotionshoes.co.uk** and **Plusinboots.co.uk.**

2. A great pair of square-heeled, round-toed boots have timeless appeal: they work well with dresses and jeans, and from day to night. Plus, they are much easier to walk in than spindly stiletto styles.

3. Re-heel and re-sole your boots every year and you will get more wear out of them.

WEAR WITH: wrap dresses, wide-hem and pencil skirts, and tucked into jeans.

STYLE NO-NO: riding boots are not great with full-on horsey clothing, like jodhpurs; they will make short legs look shorter, too.

FIND RIDING BOOTS AT: Russell & Bromley, Carvela, Kurt Geiger, Office.

• ANKLE BOOTS

THE LOOK: Short and sassy. Ankle boots have become a bit of a regular feature on the catwalks. They also come in some great mid-heel styles, so are great for any of you who are a little heel-shy. Whether you want to go for a smart look or like wearing them on casual weekender days, they will look fabulous with many of the classic looks we have covered in this book. If you don't like heels, choose a cute fringed moccasin style to wear with jeans. Or go for stiletto or platform styles for that bang-on-trend vibe.

WEAR WITH: short skirts, skinny jeans and tapered trousers.

STYLE NO-NO: wearing ankle boots with below-the-knee skirts can shorten legs; they can also make wide calves look even more so.

FIND ANKLE BOOTS AT: Office, Topshop, Dorothy Perkins, Faith.

SAVVY SAVER

IT'S EASY TO REVAMP SHOES: SO IF YOU'VE NOT WORN SOME OF YOUR OLD STYLES FOR A WHILE, WHIP THEM BACK INTO SHAPE WITH MY TOP TIPS.

1 YOU'RE SURE TO GET BORED OF SOME OF YOUR SHOES, so don't be afraid of re-colouring them. Dylon do a range of shoe-revamping products, including paints for satin, leather and synthetics. Find them at Paintsprays.co.uk.

2 REINVENT OLD COURTS AND STILETTOS IN AN INSTANT: attach a pretty corsage to the front. Or stick a velvet or satin bow to the back of the heel.

3 DESIGNER BOOTS ARE AVERAGING OUT AT AROUND £1,000 THESE DAYS, but with the high street offering some of their classiest styles in years, you should be able to find a decent quality pair for around £100–£150.

4 GET TOP DESIGNER SHOES FOR LESS: eBay is a brilliant place to find barely-worn styles by the big shoe designers, such as CHRISTIAN LOUBOUTIN and MANOLO BLAHNIK, for a fraction of the usual price.

SAVVY SHOPPER

BUYING SHOES IS ONE OF LIFE'S GREAT TREATS – HERE'S HOW TO GET THE MOST OUT OF YOUR SHOE-SHOPPING SPREES.

1 IF YOU DON'T FALL IN LOVE WITH THE SHOE ON THE SHELF, you never will – put away that purse, angel!

2 IF YOU ARE ONLY BUYING ONE PAIR, GO FOR A CLASSIC – a great stiletto will go with loads of outfits, from skinny jeans to evening dresses.

3 THEY ARE ENCRUSTED WITH JEWELS, they have seven-inch heels, and they are so fabulous that you just have to have them. Stop! Don't be tempted to buy them if you know they will only go with one dress, because they will become your new wardrobe dust-catchers.

4 PLAN SOME OUTFITS IN YOUR HEAD before you buy shoes – that way, you'll make a sensible choice.

5 DON'T ALWAYS GO FOR BLACK WHEN LOOKING AT WORK STYLES: try tan or nude for a change.

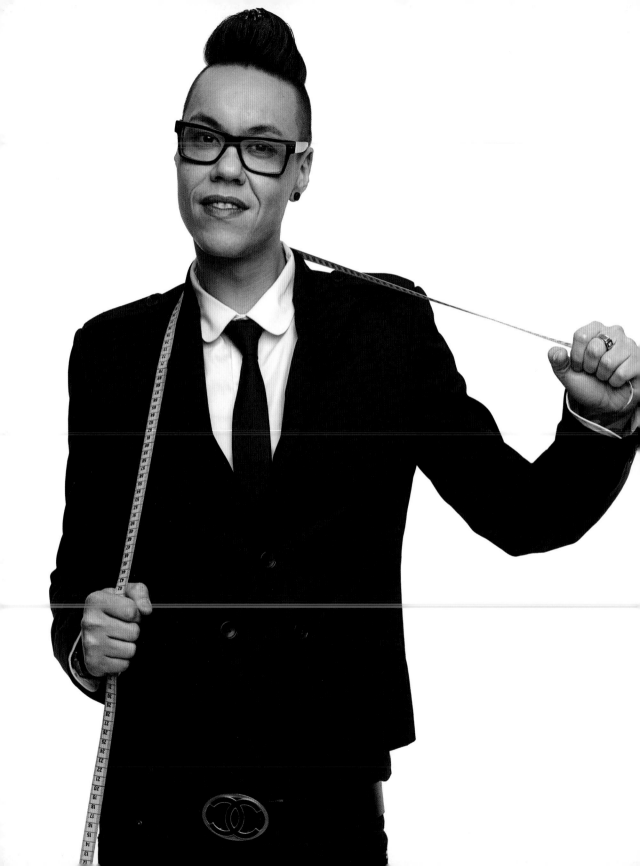

> Now you know how shoes can help you pull all the elements of your look together, girls -- and how to get more creative with them. Practical styles aside, I think every woman should make it her mission to treat herself to some real dazzlers every now and again!

jewellery

SO, LADIES, THIS IS WHERE WE START HUNTING FOR BURIED TREASURE, AND YOUR JEWELLERY BOX MARKS THE SPOT. We are going to untangle all the necklaces, earrings and other beautiful baubles you have got glittering away in there and look at how they can work to enhance your capsule looks.

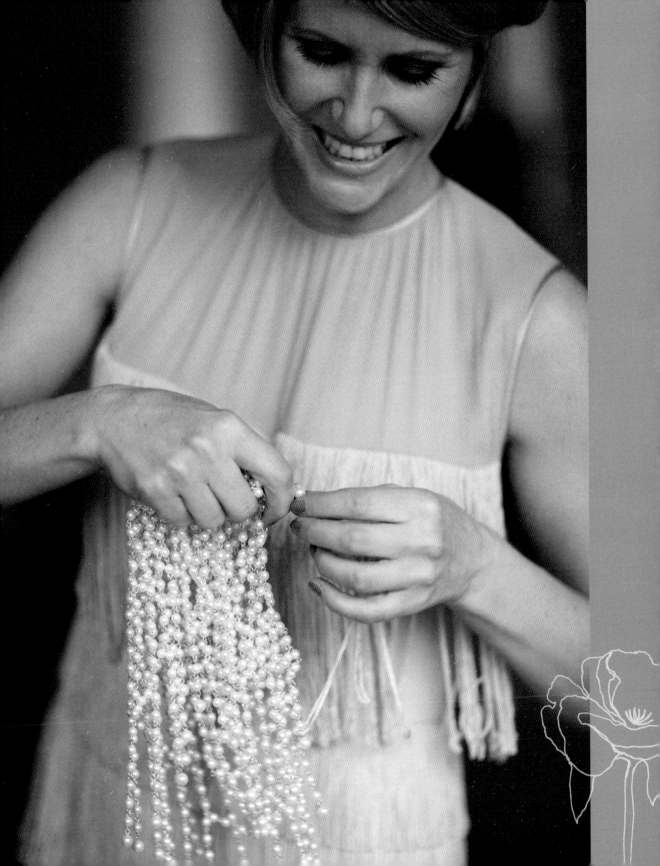

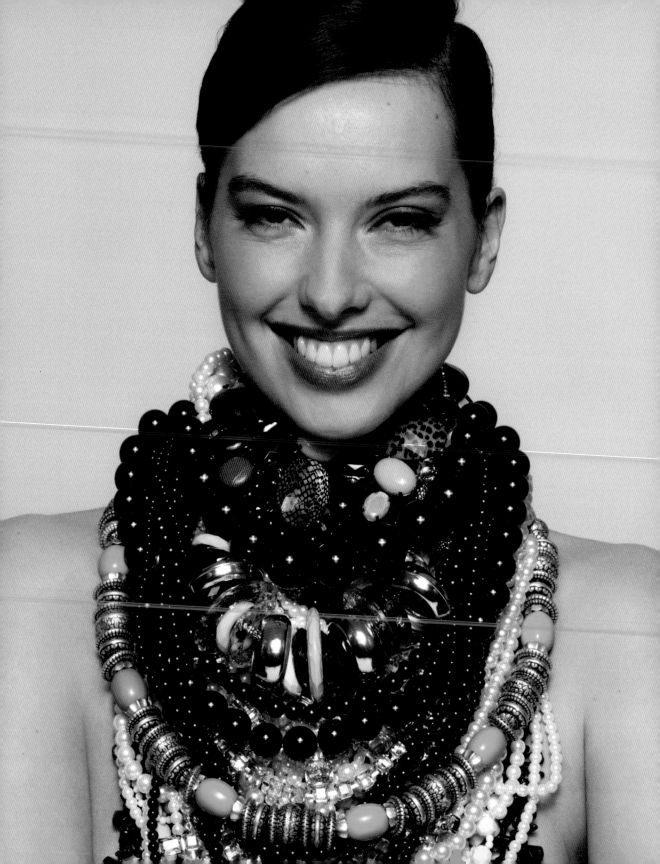

IF YOUR JEWELS HAVE LOST THEIR LUSTRE, IT COULD BE TIME TO UPDATE YOUR JEWELLERY BOX WITH SOME NEW TRINKETS. This, gorgeous, is the one area where I'd say that you can afford to treat yourself every now and again – and every girl loves a little sparkle and shine.

1.necklaces

• PEARLS

Like **Coco Chanel's No. 5 scent,** iconic tweed jacket or quilted handbag, pearls are a style classic. In fact, it was the French designer who made them the must-have item of jewellery back in the twenties. Since then, pearls have never gone out of fashion and I don't know a woman who doesn't own them in one form or other. But be careful, girls: if worn the wrong way, these little beauties can make your outfit more Miss Marple than Mademoiselle Chanel. They can be instantly ageing, and a single small, short strand is the worst culprit. Take a tip from Chanel herself and decadently wrap strings of them, in all different lengths, round your neck.

top tip

Different-length strands of pearls mixed with gilt and

jewelled chains will add a Chanel-esque touch to black outfits.

• STATEMENT NECKLACES

Big, bold, stone-encrusted neckpieces are such a hit on the catwalks now and you'll find fantastic giant necklaces to suit all occasions in most high-street stores. (Topshop, Miss Selfridge and Accessorize offer some of the best.) If you like the idea of an ethnic look, go for necklaces covered in oversized coloured stones that sit on the breastbone. Or if you're a diehard classics girl, wear a chain of giant gold links. Whatever look you want to pull off, my bold beauties, the idea here is to go for a look-at-me necklace that becomes the focus of your outfit — setting it against a plain neckline will always be your best bet.

top tip

Go for textured materials, such as wood, stone, brass and turquoise or amber, and wear with light summer layers: your necklace will look fabulous against a white vest.

• PENDANTS

Every girl has got some version of a pendant necklace in her accessories drawer — they go with every outfit under the sun, so you are sure to have put one on at some point. A leather, lace and enamel pendant was a real seventies hippy trend and that is the look you want to avoid here, ladies: it's for good reason that there are millions of these old-style pendants in charity shops. One of the loveliest ways to wear pendants now is to go for a long, delicate chain with small beads, stones or charms. Or, for a bolder approach, take any long gilt chain that you have in your jewellery box and attach the most juicy-hued giant jewel you can find.

160

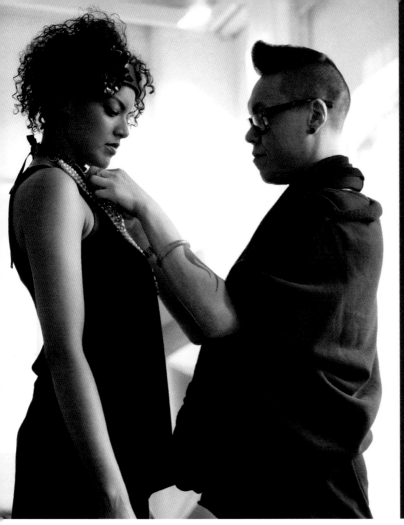
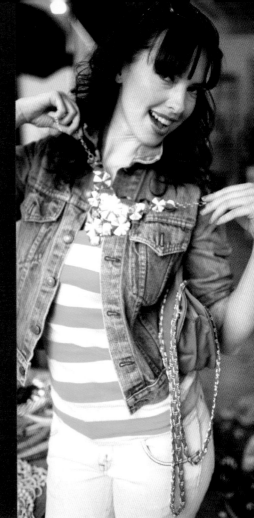

top tip

Drape your pendant over a tux -jacket and wide leg trouser combo for instant style and glam factor.

161

JEWELLERY

2.earrings

• CHANDELIER EARRINGS

They do exactly what they say on the tin, girls – hang from your ears like chandeliers. Just like the statement necklace, these supersized sparklers (some are so giant that they hang down to the shoulder or collarbone) will be the highlight of any night-time get-up. Wear with plain outfits, and keep hair swept back or away from the face to get that glitteringly glam effect.

top tip

Chandelier earrings look fabulous on longer necks. Long and dangly styles lengthen the line of the neck and slim the face. Pick up a pair now!

• STUDS AND BUTTON-STYLE

For good, everyday earrings that will work with all looks, plain gold, diamond or pearl studs are the best bet, ladies. Go for bigger versions for a more fashionable touch, and avoid wearing any of those brightly coloured plastic ones that you've had in that jewellery box since the eighties, unless a) you are going to a School Disco night, or b) you want to look like **CYNDI LAUPER** in her heyday.

• HOOPS

These are the classics of the bunch – hoops go with anything, from day to night and smart to casual. Choose medium ones for everyday and work outfits; wear giant ones on holiday with a kaftan for a hint of Moroccan summer chic and wear any of your diamond-studded or gold ones to lift office looks, Miss Nine-to-Five!

top tip

Round hoops have a lovely softening effect on square jawlines. Mid-length earrings can make shorter necks look shorter – go extra long instead!

• LONG EARRINGS

Long earrings are a super-sexy choice for evenings and glamourpusses. Avoid wearing them by day, though, as they will look too night-time and out of place.

• DELICATE EARRINGS

From pretty emerald pear drops to dangling beaded styles, delicate earrings have real classic cachet. But beware, my lovely ladies, just like pearls, old-fashioned drops can make you look just that little bit out of date. Wear with casual outfits for a more modern look.

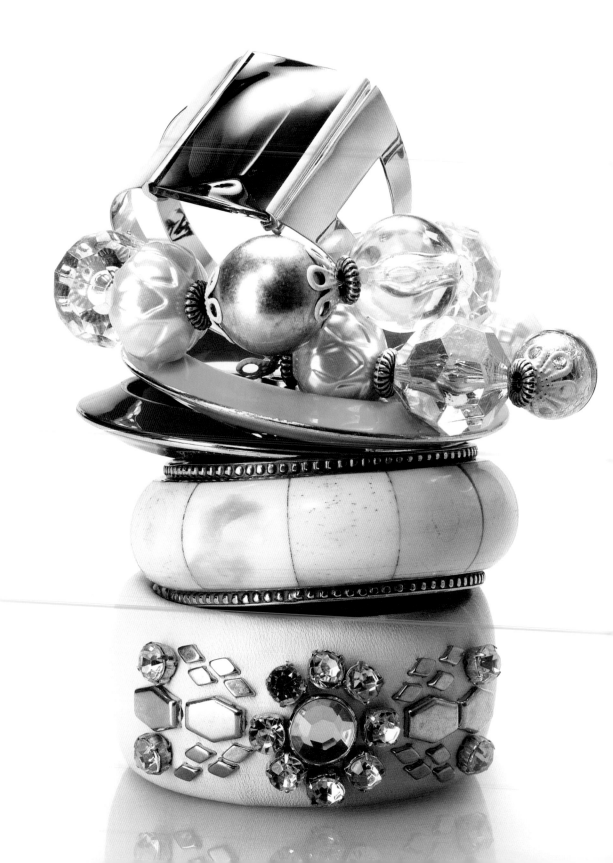

3.arm candy

HIGH-STREET ACCESSORIES DEPARTMENTS ARE JUST BRIMMING WITH FAB ARM CANDY. There are so many ways to create different looks with them, so here are just a few:

BRACELETS

- An OVERSIZED GILT-CHAIN BRACELET will give classic outfits that long-lasting Chanel-like chic. Wear with a white shirt and a pencil skirt.

- FINE CHAIN-LINK BRACELETS worn on their own work with light summer looks. They'll look good on their own with white prom-style dresses or boho maxi dresses.

BANGLES

- Wear GIANT WOODEN BANGLES in patterned designs on one arm or stack up different-sized bangles in warm colours, such as red, amber and chocolate, with black ones on both. This will add a tribal touch to a simple shirtdress.

CUFFS

- Make an entrance at evening events: wear a GIANT, GLITTERING JEWELLED CUFF with a single-sleeve dress (on the sleeved arm, not the bare one, as this will knock the look off balance).

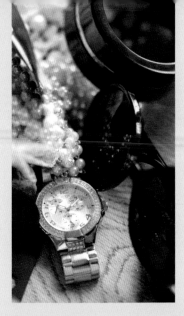

A little *word about ...*
WATCHES

YOUR WATCH IS OFTEN THE MOST PRECIOUS PIECE OF JEWELLERY YOU OWN, MY LOVELIES, BUT THAT DOESN'T MEAN TO SAY THAT YOU HAVE TO WEAR IT EVERY DAY. It's nice to change your watch (or to not wear one) to suit your look. Loads of women are now wearing oversized men's styles – they can look so cool worn loosely, like a bracelet, with a white shirt, while fine, ladylike bracelet-style cocktail watches can look quite retro in the evenings. If your granny hasn't bestowed you with one, hunt them out in those good old charity shops. If your watch is big on value – sentimental or otherwise – then don't just keep it for special occasions; enjoy wearing it more. And if you own a seriously blingy wristpiece, flash it by day or night.

166

A little word about ...
BROOCHES

A BROOCH IS A BRILLIANT WAY TO ALTER A LOOK OR CREATE A DIFFERENT KIND OF STYLE. I'd say that every jewellery box should have a big, diamanté, gemstone or jewelled brooch in it, as it's all you need to instantly lift a range of looks. If you pin a dazzling brooch to an all-black tux, it will add just the right amount of glam – you can also use it to hold you in where the jacket crosses over. This is a good tip when wearing wraparound shirts and cardigans: a brooch pinned at the crossover point at the bust can add a sweet fifties-style vibe. Glittery brooches give a real ladylike chic to daytime looks, too: pin an old jewelled brooch to a tweed jacket for that heritage back-to-the-country vibe. For an easy office-to-party update, attach two same-design brooches to either lapel of your classic black work jacket.

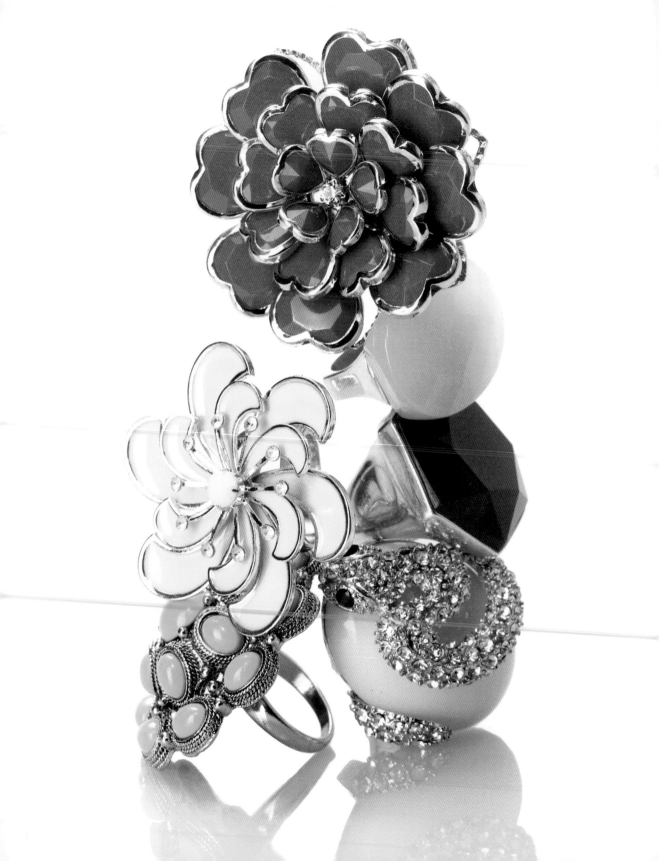

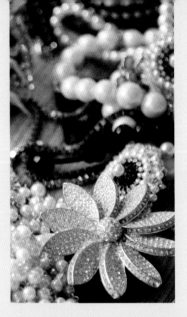

A little word about ...
RINGS

I JUST LOVE THOSE BIG, BEJEWELLED COCKTAIL RINGS THAT STORES SUCH AS ACCESSORIZE AND TOPSHOP OFFER ALL YEAR ROUND – THEY ARE SO DECADENT! And, like a fabulous brooch, one fabulous ring (it's got to be BIG) can be all you need to pep up your style. If you are wearing a dress ring, remember to take your everyday jewellery off as it will look messy and a little wrong if all worn together. For an elegant night-time look, wear one ring and no other jewellery, or slip two rings on the same hand for a more edgy take. Don't be afraid to wear these bold beauties during the day: a statement ring is an oh-so-chic addition to casual, everyday jeans-and-tee combos.

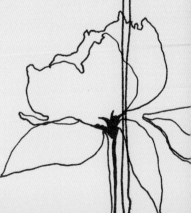

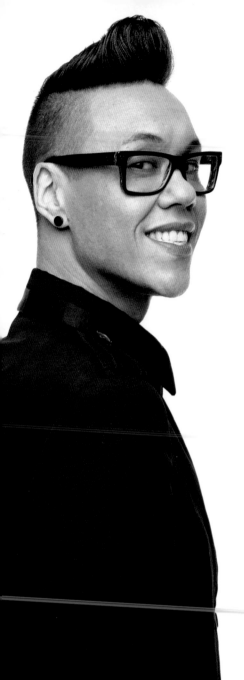

Gok's
jewel rules

Make sure your jewels are making you sparkle. Here's how:

1. BOLD AND BEAUTIFUL

If you are wearing a statement necklace or earrings, then keep all other jewellery to a minimum — these bejewelled beauties will do all the talking.

2. SILVER AND GOLD

Don't be afraid to mix gold and silver — it's a great way of getting new use out of the old chains and bracelets that have been tangled up at the bottom of your jewellery box.

3. SO CHARMING

Whether it's that simple silver chain that you got for your 21st or a classic gold-link necklace, if you've not worn it for ages, update it by threading some treasured charms or old rings on to it for really personalised style.

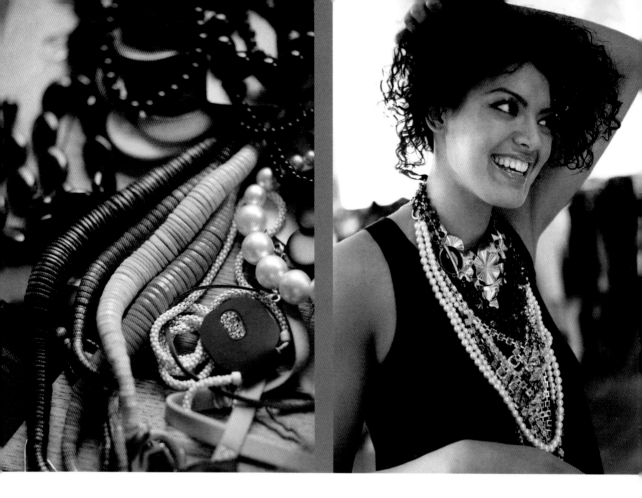

4.COLOUR CODING

For a chic evening look, choose jewels that are the same colour as your outfit – think jet stones on black, coral earrings with a coral dress and pearls on pearly satin.

5.MORE IS MORE

For instant designer style, pile on as many necklaces as you dare – you'll look bang on-trend.

171

JEWELLERY

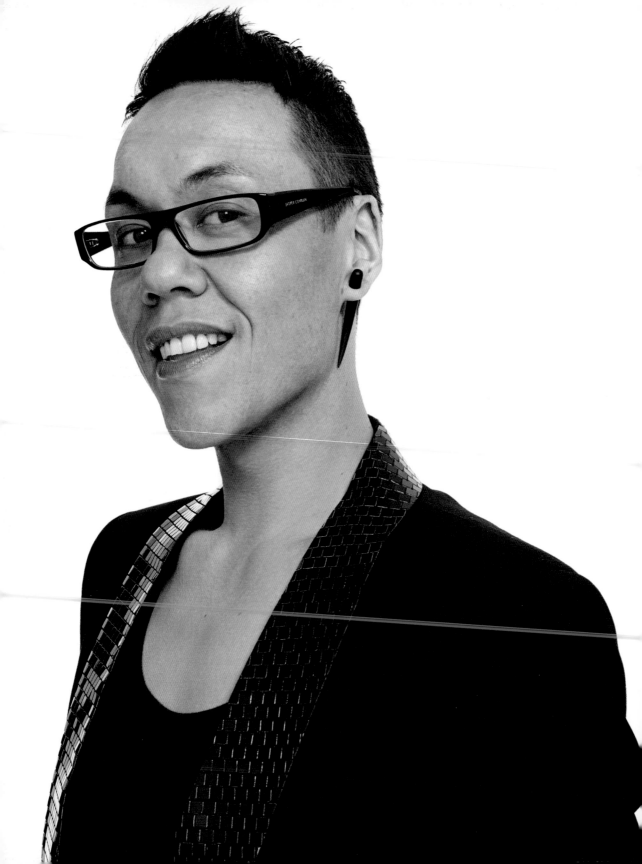

"

So, ladies, I hope you have had a good old rummage in that jewellery box. Discovered a lot of buried treasure glistening away in there? It's all you need to add a lovely, personal touch to your style. Shine on, my gorgeous girls!

"

bags, belts & scarves

YOU'VE GOT YOUR OUTFIT AND SHOES IN CHECK, ADDED A SPRINKLE OF SPARKLE, and now, my super-stylish señoritas, it's time to add the delectable details.

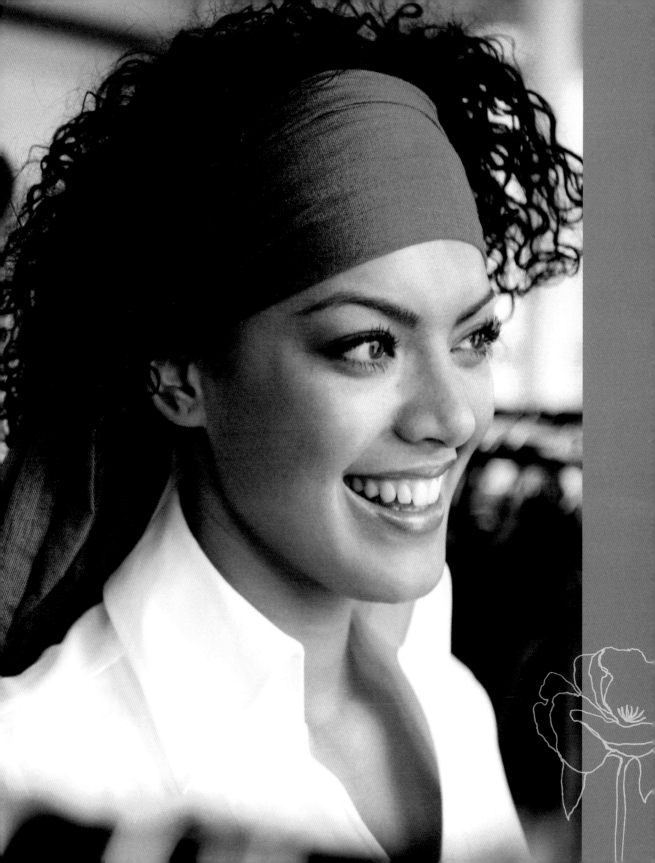

WHETHER IT'S A HEAVENLY HANDBAG, A SUMPTUOUS SILK SCARF OR A PAIR OF SUPER-GLAM SUNGLASSES, THE ACCESSORIES IN THIS CHAPTER WILL BRING YOUR OUTFIT TOGETHER AND ADD POLISH TO YOUR LOOK. These elegant extras are the easiest, most economical way to modernise any outmoded outfit and get right to the heart of credit-crunch couture. So, if you are looking for a belt to hone in on that hourglass waist, a great pair of gloves to bring that classic winter coat up to date or a cool little hat to liven up autumn looks, then, gorgeous, read on.

1.handbags

WHEN IT COMES TO OVERSTUFFED WARDROBES, MANY OF MY GIRLS HOARD HANDBAGS LIKE THEY ARE GOING OUT OF FASHION. My advice? If you haven't pulled it out in the past year, it's time to bin the baggage and bang it on the Oxfam pile. Paring down your handbag options to three key styles will not only slim down your wardrobe, but your style will get a sleeker, simpler touch, too.
TO GET YOU STARTED...

• EVERYDAY STYLES

Like that everlasting winter coat, ladies, a classic handbag should have staying power. You should be able to use it every day, carry it from day to night and sling it over your shoulder at weekends. Anything big, simple and slouchy in black, brown or tan leather will look good year after year and will go with pretty much anything. (Brown and tan tones work well with softer summer colours.) A good handbag should work just as well with jeans as it does with a smart office look and will hold all your daily essentials – even the kitchen sink if required. (I know how much you girls carry in there!)

where to buy

STYLE BUY: Topshop, Warehouse, ASOS, Next, Miss Selfridge, New Look, John Lewis **INVESTMENT BUY:** TK Maxx, Jaeger, Gap, Mulberry, Theoutnet.com, M&S, Kipling, Zara, Coccinelle, Net-a-porter.com, Hobbs

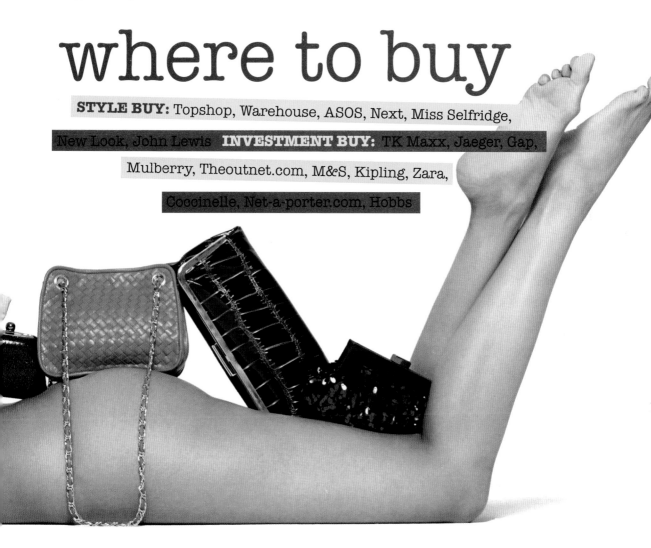

• STATEMENT STYLES

One of the easiest ways to add a modern edge to any classic outfit is to offset its simplicity with a bag that's big on 'wow' factor. While many statement bags tend to be quite big in size, some are just big in character, like super-trendy studded ones, or those with lots of gold buckles and straps. Brightly coloured bags are also a great way to make a style statement: a huge red patent tote will really sass up a plain polo-neck and capri-pants combo, for instance.

where to buy

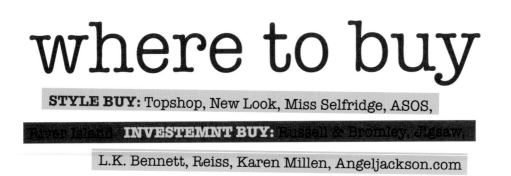

STYLE BUY: Topshop, New Look, Miss Selfridge, ASOS, River Island. **INVESTEMNT BUY:** Russell & Bromley, Jigsaw, L.K. Bennett, Reiss, Karen Millen, Angeljackson.com

• OCCASION STYLES

Because you don't use them every day, your evening bags should always be a little bit special and a whole lot glam – the final addition that makes you know you are red-carpet ready. A lovely evening bag can work like an amazing piece of jewellery. So, if you like the idea of night-time sparkle, go for the most shimmery evening bag you can find. Or, if you don't want your bag to clash with your outfit too much, go for a simple clutch in a luxe fabric, such as black satin or velvet. A brightly coloured evening bag will look amazing with that LBD.

178

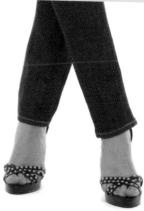

where to buy

STYLE BUY: Faith, Accessorize, Monsoon, Dune, Red Herring at Debenhams **INVESTMENT BUY:** L.K. Bennett, Karen Millen, Angeljackson.com, Mulberry, Marc by Marc Jacobs, Reiss

179

BAGS, BELTS AND SCARVES

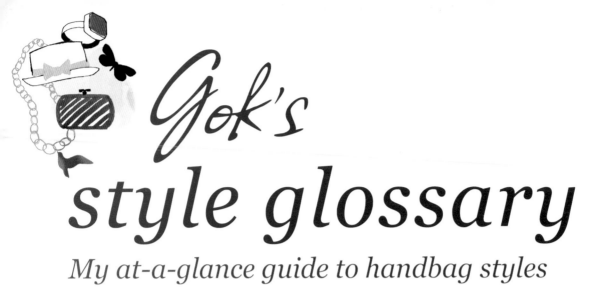

Gok's style glossary

My at-a-glance guide to handbag styles

- **TOTE:** a big, roomy bag that is perfect for casual looks – and shopping!

- **SHOULDER BAG:** a medium-sized, smartish everyday option.

- **OVERSIZED:** it makes a giant statement and offsets simple get-ups well.

- **GIANT CLUTCH:** a big, super-cool leather envelope style will add a trendy edge to daytime looks.

- **EVENING CLUTCH:** soft or structured, and big enough to carry a lipstick and mirror. An opulent clasp will up the glam factor on this little beauty.

- **EVENING SHOULDER BAG:** for those who don't like to carry their bag in their hand all night and who like a little more room, this smallish style with pretty detailed straps is the perfect choice.

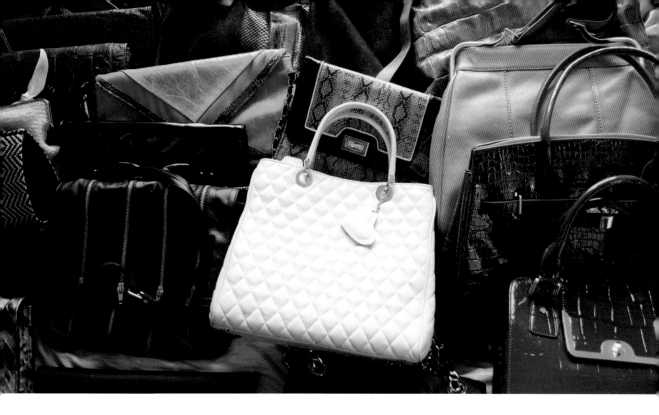

BUYING TIP...

Although I love the great choice of high-street hold-alls, it's only a small section of styles that are made well enough to stay the course. If it's a do-all classic you're after, you'll need to splash out a little on an investment buy – a good-quality leather handbag will prove its style credentials year after year and develop that gorgeous love-worn look.

181

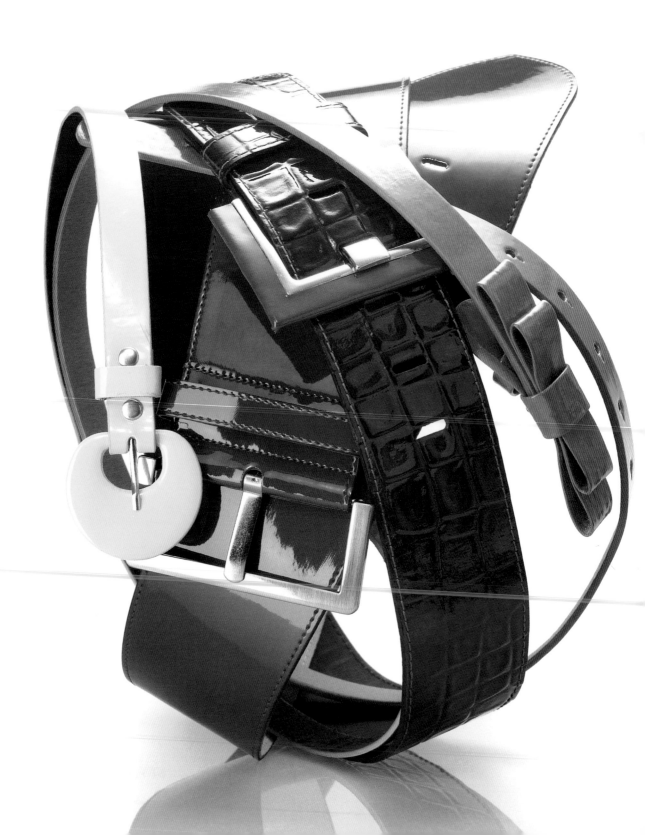

2.belts

IF THERE'S ONE THING I'D SAY YOU CAN NEVER, EVER HAVE ENOUGH OF, LADIES, IT'S BELTS. They are such a brilliant style all-rounder: they can transform your shape, add instant cool to casual outfits and smarten up any style. Medium-size tan, black and brown leather ones always look best with denims and cords. Brightly coloured skinny ones add a kooky touch to skinny black or coloured jeans and can add a super-stylish edge to plain shift dresses or wrapped round plain wool cardies. Big, opulent buckles will draw attention to your waist and make a statement by day or night (they look so glam when worn with maxi dresses), while wide waist-cinchers can add a sexy fifties look to pencil and prom skirts.

where to buy

STYLE BUY: Topshop, New Look, M&S, ASOS, Next, John Lewis

INVESTMENT BUY: Ted Baker, Reiss, Mulberry, Dorothy Perkins, Jaeger

Stephencollins.co.uk, House of Fraser. Net-a-porter.com

183

3.scarves

THERE IS NO LIMIT TO WHAT YOU CAN DO WITH SCARVES AND I JUST LOVE THE WAY THAT THEY'VE BECOME SUCH A KEY PART OF FASHION LOOKS. There are so many great ways for upping the style factor with a scarf. Here are just a few:

1.CARRIED AWAY

Add a glam touch to your everyday casual bag by tying a small printed silk scarf round the end of one of the handles.

2.THE HOLIDAY WRAP

Fold your scarf over once into a triangle, put your head forward, gather the scarf round the back of the neck, then keep twisting the fabric at the front until you have one length. Throw it over your head and you have a super-glam turban that makes an ideal holiday hat!

3.THE BELT-UP

Take a large, square scarf, fold the ends in to the middle (as if you were wrapping a parcel), then twist it into a long length of fabric and use it as a belt. Wear it round a white shirt, loop it through your jeans or belt up your mac with it.

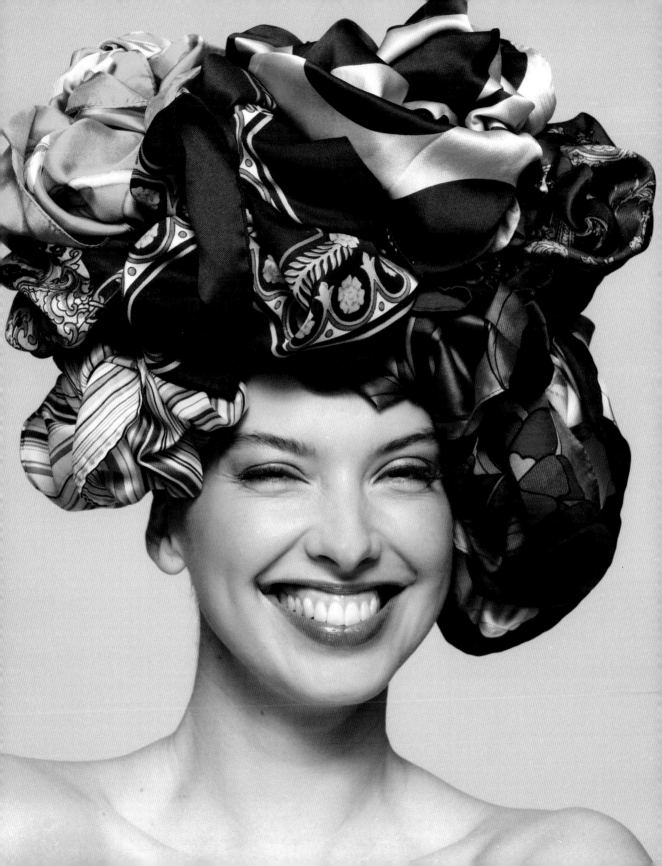

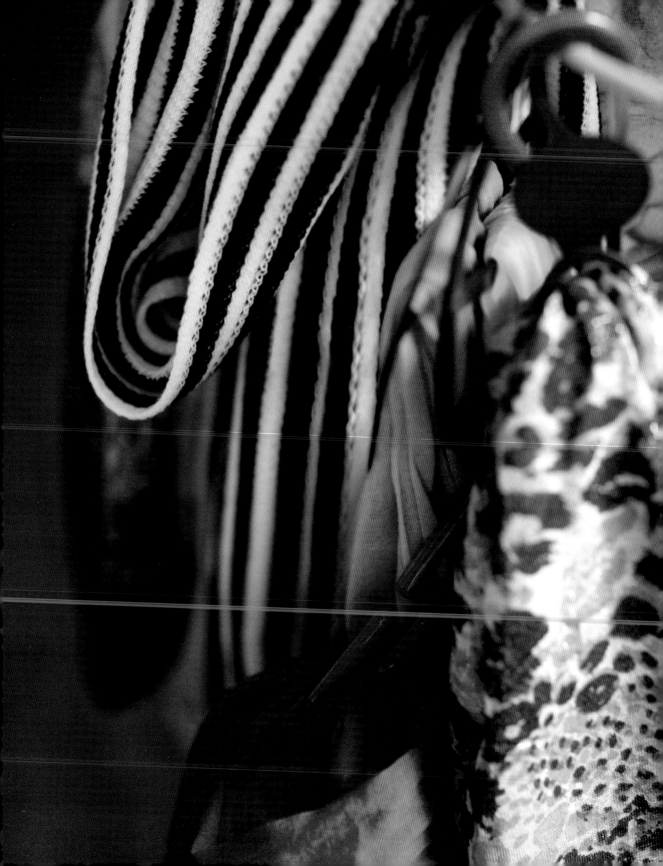

> **Don't fold your pashmina into a triangle over your shoulders unless fortune-teller chic is a look you love.**

4.ELEGANTLY EXOTIC

Animal-print or metallic scarves add a hint of glam to daytime get-ups. In the evening, choose long, skinny chiffon styles for old-style glamour.

5.THE CHIC WRAP

The best way to wear really big scarves is to loop them loosely round your neck: a casually draped big, printed cotton or fine wool scarf will add a gorgeously chic touch to off-duty looks.

6.THE PARISIAN TOUCH

For a more sophisticated, preppy take, tie a small, silky scarf closely round your neck, and add a final flourish by knotting it.

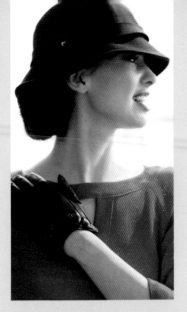

A little word about ...
HATS

THEY DO CROP UP ON THE CATWALKS EVERY NOW AND AGAIN, BUT I'M STILL WAITING FOR THE DAY WHEN HATS MAKE A HUGE COMEBACK. I love hats and I think every single woman should wear a hat at some point, and not just to a wedding. There's something empowering about wearing a hat as part of an everyday look. A classic fedora, for instance, looks super-sassy when worn with city shorts and a blazer, while a little Breton cap – like the ones that sailors used to wear – looks cute in autumn worn with a stripy top or a winter coat. The beret is, of course, the most classic fashion hat of all – it's the perfect accompaniment to your mac and works as a chic cover-up for those bad-hair days. If you think that hats are not your bag, ladies, go on, just try some on. You will be pleasantly surprised.

188

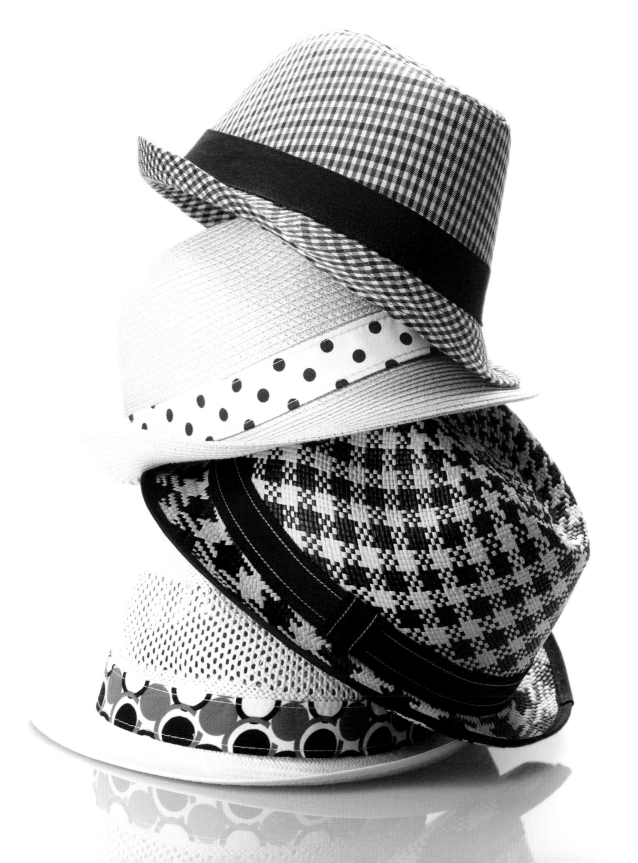

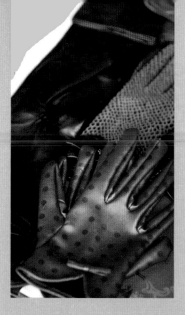

A little *word* about ...
GLOVES

APART FROM KEEPING YOUR HANDS WARM IN WINTER, YOU CAN GET QUITE CREATIVE WITH DIFFERENT GLOVE STYLES. In summer, dayglo lacy or net ones can heighten the prettiness of summer dresses – it's a look that **LILY ALLEN** can pull off well; brightly hued leather gloves (John Lewis do the most fabulous selection) can add an elegant swathe of colour to dark winter coats; and long leather gloves can look fab when worn with a tux (push the sleeves up to the elbow at night). While it used to be a favourite party look in the eighties, these days long satin gloves can look a little old-fashioned with evening dresses (so wear a giant cocktail ring instead).

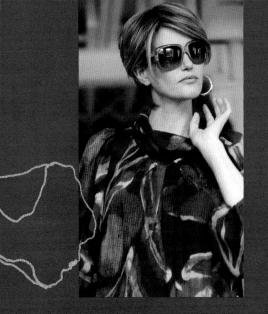

A little word about ...
SUNGLASSES

JUST LIKE SHOES, THERE ARE NO AGE RESTRICTIONS, NO FIGURE RESTRAINTS AND NO LIMITS TO HOW GLAM YOU WANT TO GO – SUNGLASSES ARE JUST THE MOST FAB ACCESSORY EVER! Whether you are jetting off to Ibiza, popping out for a pint of milk on a Sunday morning or avoiding the paparazzi, nothing makes you feel more like a superstar than a pair of super-cool sunnies. If statement sunglasses say too much for you, go for classic shapes, such as Ray-Ban Aviators or Wayfarers (both have had a real renaissance of late), which will last you for years. Just remember to make sure that whichever pair you buy have lenses designed to protect your eyes from the sun.

191

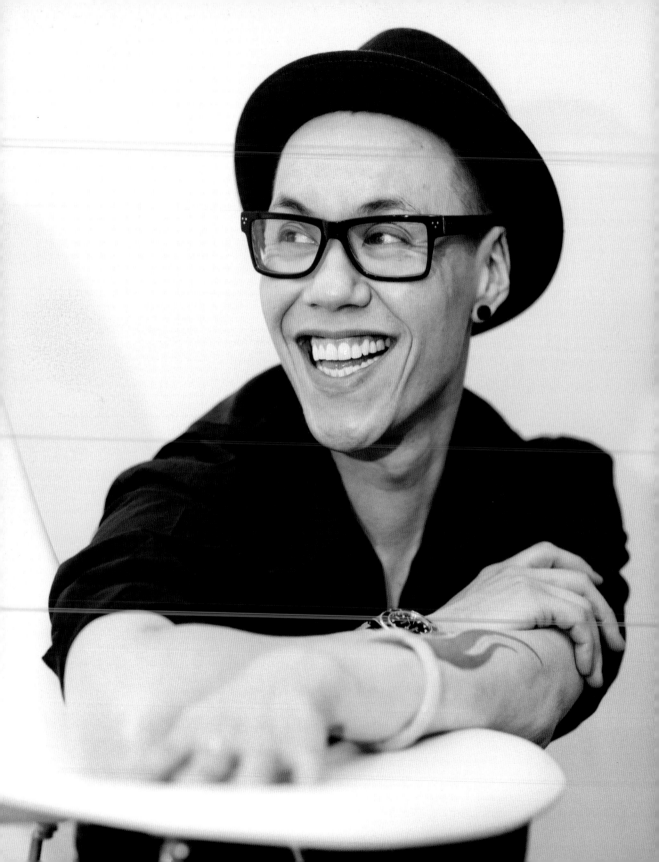

> However far you want to go with your accessories, my darlings, use these fabulous fashion accents to really personalise your look: they will say everything you want to about your sensational style.

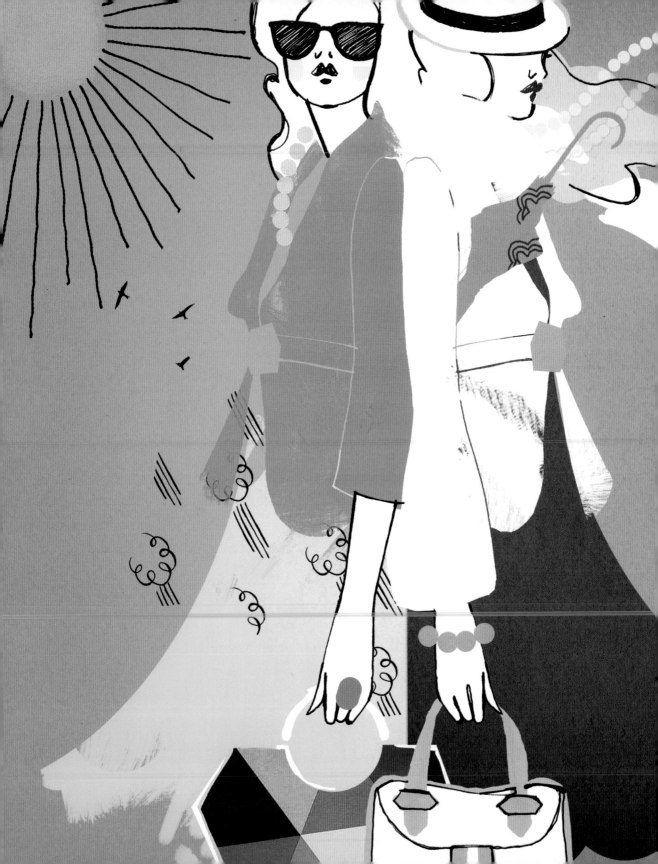

timeless style

We all know that fashions come and go, but some trends never, ever date. Here's my guide to everlasting seasonal style

trends

spring/ summer

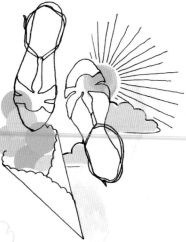

THE DAYS ARE LONGER, THE SUN SHINES, AND EVERYTHING FEELS LIGHTER AND BRIGHTER. LADIES, there's nothing like the new spring/summer season to put you in the mood for spring-cleaning your wardrobe and giving it a fresh fashion boost.

> 66
>
> *From now on, stylish summer dressing will be a breeze.*
>
> 99

THERE'S NO DOUBT THAT YOU'LL HAVE TO UPDATE YOUR WARDROBE with a few new pieces to suit the warmer months. But as you already have the basics in check – whether it's your white shirt, your floral dress or a classic blazer – this chapter is all about looking at how to style them up to create classic trends with staying power. **Here are FIVE TIMELESS LOOKS for SPRING/SUMMER:**

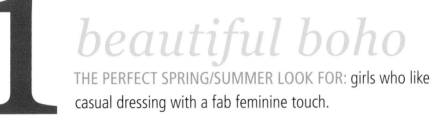

1 *beautiful boho*

THE PERFECT SPRING/SUMMER LOOK FOR: girls who like casual dressing with a fab feminine touch.

GOK'S STYLE GLOSSARY: the essence of any boho look is to mix colours, patterns and textures.

GET THE LOOK: There are many ways to do boho now, ladies, but basically, the style rule here is to **mix but don't match!** So you might wear one of your floral tunic dresses with some gladiator sandals and some hippy-style accessories.

ESSENTIAL EXTRAS: tribal or ethnic-style jewellery is essential to the boho look. Think leather fringing, stacks of bangles and huge statement necklaces.

GOK'S STYLE TIP: more is more here, so don't be afraid to pile on accessories. Or just add boho-style elements, such as an embroidered top, and wear with jeans.

SHOP THE LOOK: Next, Per Una at M&S, Day Birger et Mikkelsen.

WORKING THE LOOK: Kate Moss, Sienna Miller, Alexa Chung and Twiggy.

Don't hold back on the accessories, girls – go on, pile them on!

Gladiator sandals are the perfect way to update the hippy-chic look.

199

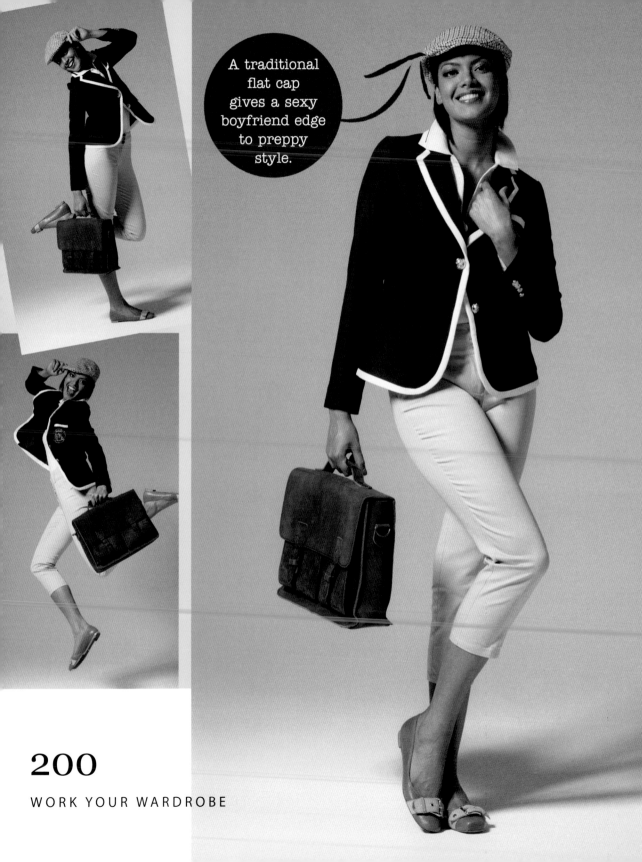

A traditional flat cap gives a sexy boyfriend edge to preppy style.

2 *pretty preppy*

THE PERFECT SPRING/SUMMER LOOK FOR: anyone who likes everyday smart-casual looks.

GOK'S STYLE GLOSSARY: this crisp, clean and boyish style is understated and neat.

GET THE LOOK: this is where those chinos or capri pants come in – neat-fitting trousers are a good base for the preppy look, though any of your plain wide skirts or white skinny jeans will look great, too. Pair with a crisp white shirt or a polo shirt and slip a blazer or your mac on top. Flat shoes are the classic option – brogues, loafers or plimsolls will work – but a natural-toned wedge sandal will add to the classic feel and the height will streamline your shape.

ESSENTIAL EXTRAS: just sling on your everyday handbag in a neutral shade, classic pearl earrings and necklace (short single strands only – this look is all about conservative cool).

GOK'S STYLE TIP: a traditional flat cap will give the look fabulous flair and a sexy boyfriend-style touch.

SHOP THE LOOK: Gap, M&S, Uniqlo, Littlewoods Direct, Next, Reiss.

WORKING THE LOOK: Kate Hudson, Jennifer Aniston, Alexa Chung and Carla Bruni.

201

3 *brilliant black and white*

THE PERFECT SPRING/SUMMER LOOK FOR: girls who want to look hot in the city all summer long.

GOK'S STYLE GLOSSARY: this magic monochrome combination adds a shade of smartness to summer styles.

GET THE LOOK: black-and-white combinations have a real uptown feel and it's a sleek style that looks just as good in the office as it does for weekend lunch dates. It's smart and a little sexy, too. Wear a black cotton pencil skirt (keep legs bare) or capri pants with a plain white shirt or vest and pair with black ballet pumps and some fine gold chains for a chic day look. Or wear a printed black-and-white prom dress or wide skirt with a plain black T-shirt. A simple black and white shift dress will look great with pretty white accessories.

ESSENTIAL EXTRAS: black and white accessories are best. A structured retro-style bag will look sensational. Giant black or white sunnies will give you that cool city edge.

GOK'S STYLE TIP: black-and-white summer combos work best on sun-kissed skin, so if you're milky-white, top up the self-tanner for a golden glow.

SHOP THE LOOK: M&S, Debenhams, Gap, Next, Dorothy Perkins, Banana Republic.

WORKING THE LOOK: Sharon Stone, Katie Holmes, Helen Mirren, Kate Moss and Kylie Minogue.

202

A simple black shift dress with a white collar is the easy way to do black and white.

Perfect for everyday looks, pretty bow-front pumps are smart and stylish.

203

Silver and gold accessories look beautifully elegant with nude tones.

4 *second skin*

THE PERFECT SPRING/SUMMER LOOK FOR: on-trend girls who love to flaunt their fabulous figures.

GOK'S STYLE GLOSSARY: a subtly sexy look defined by body-skimming fabrics in soft, nude tones.

GET THE LOOK: although at first it may seem like a look that very few girls can pull off, all it takes to work this is a little shape know-how. Go for a clingy sheath dress or skirt in a silky jersey fabric in a pinkish blush or a nude tone. (Avoid anything too beige or peachy, as some shades are often not subtle or soft enough.) If you don't want to show off too much, wear one of your fine-knit cardigans over the dress and clasp with a skinny belt, or go for a clingy skirt only and drape loose layers on top (using a white vest as a starting point).

ESSENTIAL EXTRAS: gold and silver jewellery will add punch to neutral tones, as will gold gladiator sandals or heels. Wear nude stilettos for a polished look.

GOK'S STYLE TIP: this is essentially a softly tailored style, so opt for dresses, trousers and tops in fluid jersey fabric, or with ruffles and gently ruched detail. Navy complements nude shades more than black. This is also a fab look for dark skins; paler complexions could look a little washed out.

SHOP THE LOOK: Reiss, H&M, Topshop, ASOS, Firetrap.

WORKING THE LOOK: Scarlett Johannson, Angelina Jolie, Cheryl Cole and Jennifer Lopez.

205

5 *fabulous florals*

THE PERFECT SPRING/SUMMER LOOK FOR: ladies who love rocking romantic looks.

GOK'S STYLE GLOSSARY: soft, feminine and oh-so-pretty, florals never go out of fashion with designers – or fashion lovers.

GET THE LOOK: if you've got great legs, go for a short tulip-style skirt in a medium floral print and wear it with your simple white vest and some flat thong sandals. Or go for a chiffon maxi dress with big painterly splashes of pastel-coloured florals and cinch at the waist with a wide tan leather belt. If you are more of a hip kid, choose a giant single flower-print on a mini shift dress. Or simply pull out your prom dress and slip a print cardigan on top. Jackets with floral linings are a nice way to give a hint of floral print to outfits – just roll up the sleeves. If you're a real jeans girl then pair them with the most fabulous floral-print shirt you can find.

ESSENTIAL EXTRAS: there's a lot going on with floral prints, so you can keep bold accessories to a minimum. Dainty gilt chains will heighten the prettiness of this look, and hoop earrings will work, too.

GOK'S STYLE TIP: short denim and leather jackets add a hip edge to florals and stop them looking twee.

SHOP THE LOOK: French Connection, ASOS, Dorothy Perkins, Luella, Kate Moss at Topshop.

WORKING THE LOOK: Cheryl Cole, Kirsten Dunst and Lily Allen.

Florals don't always come in spriggy patterns: big prints add drama.

Don't always opt for black accessories – softer shades work best in summer.

208

WORK YOUR WARDROBE

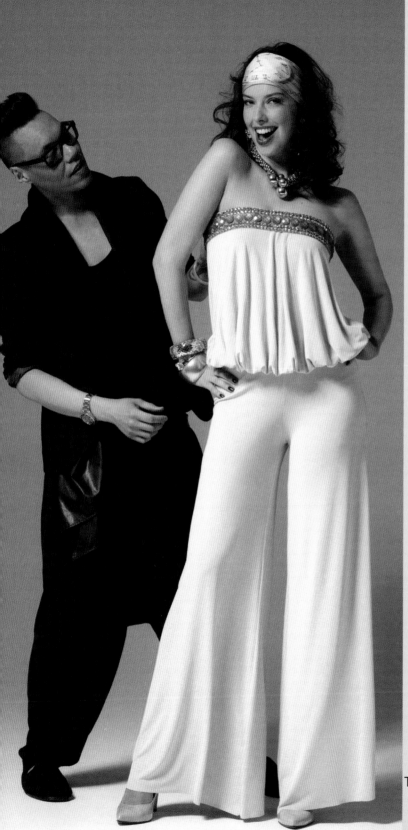

> "It's summer, girlfriend, and you have all it takes to look hot, hot, hot."

TRENDS: SPRING/SUMMER

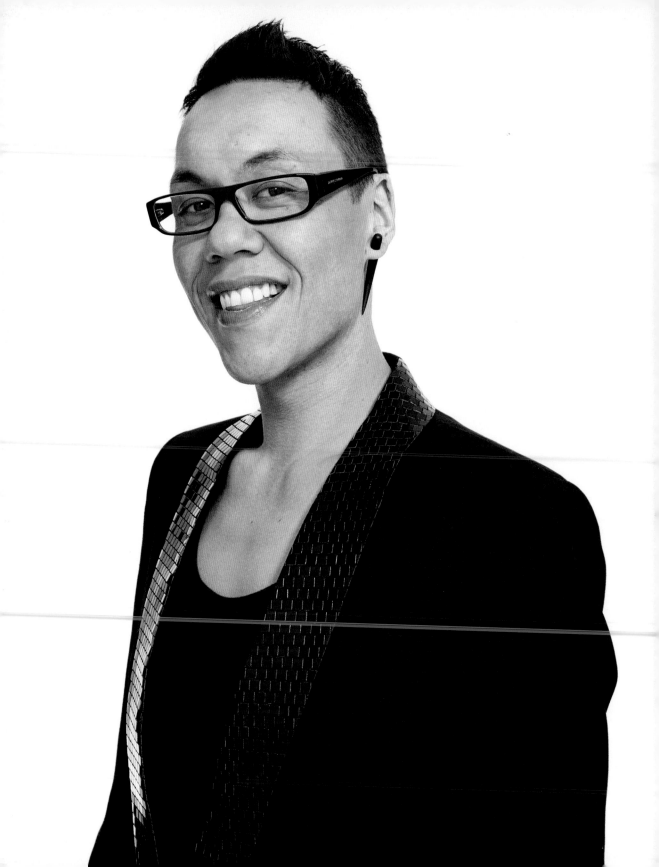

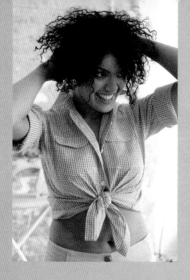

A little word about ...
SUMMER COLOUR

THE CHANGE FROM ONE SEASON TO THE NEXT IS ALWAYS TRICKY, AND AFTER BEING SERIOUSLY SWATHED IN DARK, COSY CLOTHING ALL WINTER (THOUGH WHO'S COMPLAINING?), THE IDEA OF INTRODUCING SOME LIGHTER, BRIGHTER COLOURS INTO YOUR SPRING STYLE IS AS REJUVENATING AS IT IS REFRESHING. If you've got black, dark or olive skin, the switch to colour is relatively easy because – whether pale pink or vibrant orange – vibrant shades look amazing on you lovelies. All my pale angels, however, may find that some shades make you feel a little washed out. If that rings a bell with you, then I'd suggest you layer pastel colours with tonal shades such as navy and grey (black can look way too harsh at this time of year), so you might wear a coral vest top with a navy cardigan.

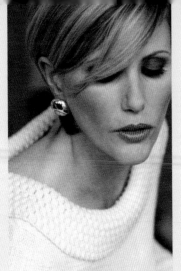

A little word about ...
SUMMER SKIN

AS THE LONG, HOT DAYS AND BALMY NIGHTS BREEZE IN, YOU'LL WANT TO WEAR LESS, BUT, LADIES, WHETHER YOU ARE A PETITE TWENTY-YEAR-OLD OR A FABULOUS FORTYSOMETHING, IT'S WORTH THINKING ABOUT HOW MUCH YOU DARE TO BARE. There aren't many girls who look their best with a naked midriff exposed – even Britney is covering up hers these days. There are more subtle ways to reveal summer skin: button down your shirt to reveal a lovely expanse of neck, or wear T-shirts with short, flouncy sleeves so that most of your arm is on show. Minis will look best halfway down the thigh and no higher, and city shorts look really sexy against bare sun-kissed legs in summer. At night, sleeveless long or short dresses look sensational.

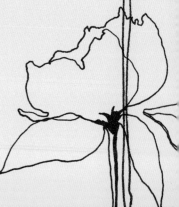

212

*A little **word** about ...*

PREPARING YOUR WARDROBE FOR SUMMER

IF YOU MAKE ROOM FOR YOUR SUMMER WARDROBE, IT WILL BE EASIER TO SEE YOUR SEPARATES AND TO PUT OUTFITS TOGETHER. Start by packing away all the winter essentials that you won't be needing for a while, such as heavy coats and jumpers, hats, gloves, winter boots and woolly tights, and store them carefully in sealed storage bags. (Go to www.johnlewis.com for a great selection.) Cotton vests and light tops can look tatty after a year, so consider whether you'll wear them again. Then take a look at everything else you have hanging in there and be as ruthless as you can before hitting the charity shops with all that closet clutter. If you've lost or put on weight, don't be tempted to hang on to things with a view to fitting into them at some point: dress for the way you are now – gorgeous.

213

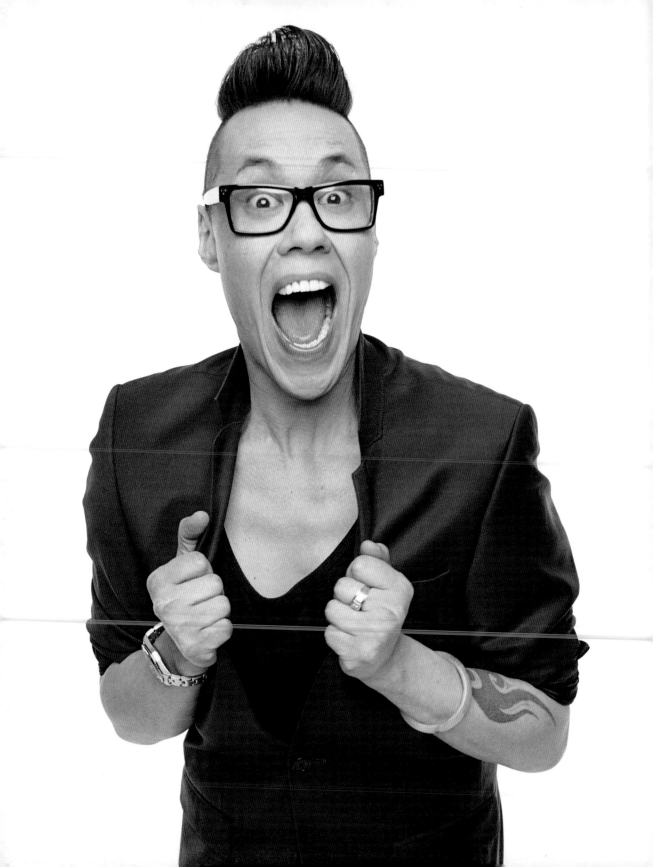

> Whether you are jetting off to sunnier climes or just hanging out at home, you've got your entire summer kit in the bag. So when the rays start to shine, all that you have to do, my sun-kissed sensations, is go out and have some fashion fun in the sun.

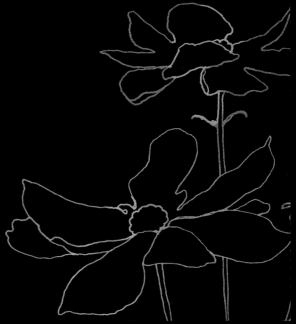

trends
autumn/
winter

THE LEAVES ARE FALLING, THE NIGHTS ARE DRAWING IN, AND THERE'S A DEFINITE NIP IN THE AIR. Yes, my snow queens, it's time to start wrapping up, unwrapping your winter wardrobe and thinking about some great new looks. After all, there's nothing like a seasonal fashion fix to cheer up darker days.

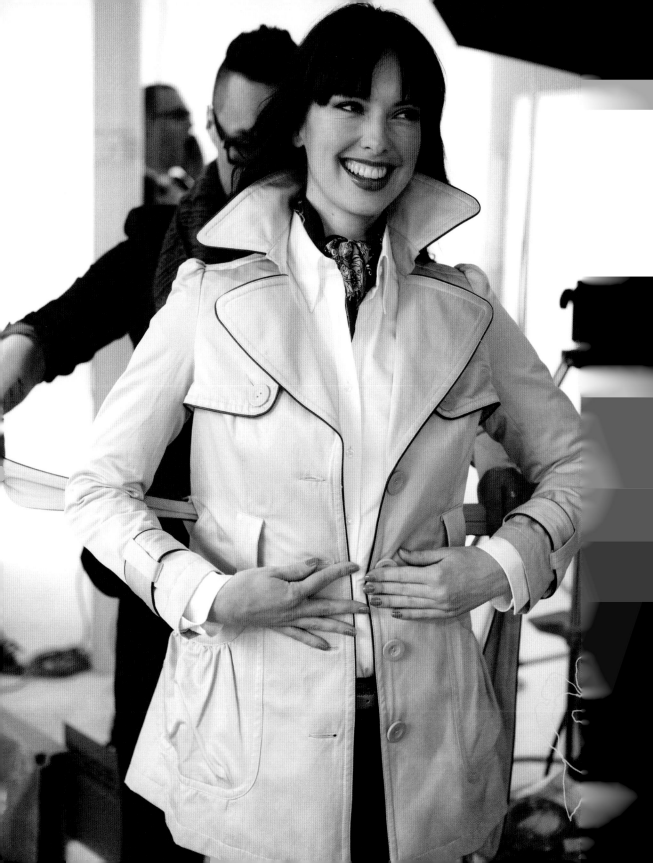

FROM GETTING THE WARMTH FACTOR RIGHT TO LOOKING CHIC DURING AUTUMN SHOWERS, in this chapter we'll work with your basics to create a set of styles that will be bang on-trend whatever the weather. I'll also take you through some glitteringly gorgeous evening looks that will make you shine the whole season through. HERE ARE FIVE TIMELESS LOOKS FOR AUTUMN/WINTER:

1 *military mode*

THE PERFECT AUTUMN/WINTER LOOK FOR: girls who like to keep it super-smart with a chic edge.

GOK'S STYLE GLOSSARY: these sharply tailored uniform-inspired styles are defined by military detailing, such as gilt buttons and frogging.

GET THE LOOK: pick a military style jacket and wear with your classic black trousers and a loose knit woollen scarf in a contrasting colour.

ESSENTIAL EXTRAS: a patent leather bag with gold or brass buckles and studs will add to the military vibe, as will a pair of long leather gloves.

GOK'S STYLE TIP: for a really chic take on this look, sling your military-style jacket over a long, silky evening dress for a glam (and warm!) night out.

SHOP THE LOOK: ASOS, Topshop, Debenhams, House of Fraser, Primark.

WORKING THE LOOK: Beyoncé, Kate Moss, Rihanna, Sienna Miller and Fearne Cotton.

Look for uniform-inspired detailing like frogging and brass buttons.

Update the military look with some on-trend mannish brogues.

219

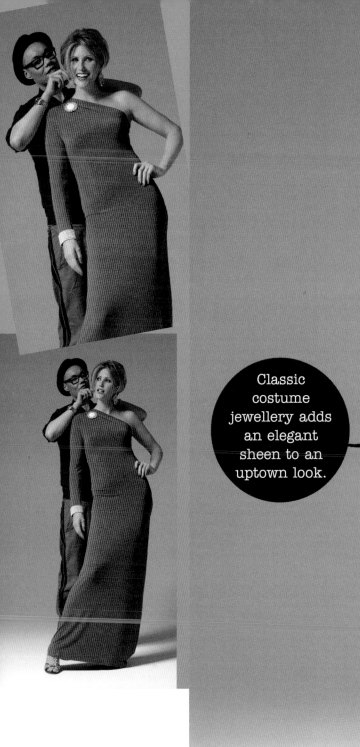

Classic costume jewellery adds an elegant sheen to an uptown look.

WORK YOUR WARDROBE

2 *glamorous gowns*

THE PERFECT AUTUMN/WINTER LOOK FOR: those who like the idea of adding real red-carpet glamour to special occasions.

GOK'S STYLE GLOSSARY: floor-skimming dresses inspired by vintage Hollywood style will always be in fashion.

GET THE LOOK: this extra-special party look is sophisticated and super-glam. Go for the slinkiest, figure-hugging fabric in the boldest shade you can find and wear with 'look-at-me' attitude. An off-the-shoulder style is figure flattering as the hint of skin adds a sultry, subtle sexiness. And remember to step into those sassy open-toe stiletto sandals, sassy lady!

ESSENTIAL EXTRAS: classic costume jewellery, such as a big diamanté bracelet, adds extra sheen to glamorous gowns. You don't need to wear tights – give legs a glow with some fake tan or shimmery body lotion. Glossy nails, lips and groomed hair are a must with this look, my fabulous fashionistas!

GOK'S STYLE TIP: long dresses should skim the toes: beware of hems that are too short as they won't flatter anyone's figure.

SHOP THE LOOK: Jaeger, Karen Millen, French Connection, Reiss, DKNY.

WORKING THE LOOK: Victoria Beckham, Carla Bruni, Cate Blanchett, Michelle Obama and Catherine Zeta-Jones.

221

3 *foxy fringing*

THE PERFECT AUTUMN/WINTER LOOK FOR: girls who like a classic party look with a glamorous edge.

GOK'S STYLE GLOSSARY: taking its cue from 1920s flapper dresses, fringing has a decadently luxurious feel and is a great choice for occasion dressing.

GET THE LOOK: the brilliant thing about fringing, ladies, is that it creates an instantly strong look. And, because all those rows and rows of silky threads really shimmy while you walk, fringed garments always feel extra-special to wear. So, instead of reaching for that little black dress for your next big party, why not opt for an elegant fringed one, instead? A nude-toned style will work really well for special occasions, like a day at the races or a wedding. Or, for evening dos, wear a fringed vest top with plain black trousers or jeans: metallic-tinged fringing has an especially glam touch.

ESSENTIAL EXTRAS: a few stacked gold bracelets and plain hoop earrings will look fab.

GOK'S STYLE TIP: sleeveless or vest-style dresses and tops are the more flattering option as the slimline silhouette won't make you look too bulky.

SHOP THE LOOK: Topshop, Zara, ASOS, Debenhams.

WORKING THE LOOK: Madonna and Michelle Obama.

222

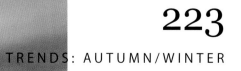

223

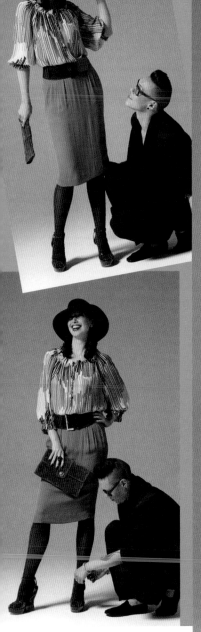

Brightly
coloured tights
are a great way
to add a funky
splash of
colour.

224

4 *clash of colour*

THE PERFECT AUTUMN/WINTER LOOK FOR: ladies looking for an edgy take on traditional winter dressing.

GOK'S STYLE GLOSSARY: this look is all about big, bold sweeps of colour cutting a sassy swathe through dark winter days.

GET THE LOOK: bright colours generally used to be associated with summer styles, but I just love the way that designers are frequently adding a punch to their winter looks by offsetting neutral winter shades, such as navy, brown and black, with vibrant bursts of colour. So you might wear a turquoise pencil skirt with a bright, stripey blouse and a purple suede belt, or you can wear a little black dress with a pair of brilliant-blue shoes. For those days when you need a lift, go for top-to-toe brights – a red skirt suit will brighten up any winter's day. Or wear a bright-pink or tomato-red coat or jacket. Colour is an instant mood-booster.

ESSENTIAL EXTRAS: accessories the same colour as the top you are wearing give outfits a really chic edge. So if you are wearing a yellow top, go for a yellow necklace. If you are wearing a black top, go for black necklaces – don't feel you always have to offset one garment with accessories in a contrasting shade.

GOK'S STYLE TIP: brightly coloured tights are the most economical way to add a funky splash of colour to all-black styles.

SHOP THE LOOK: ASOS, La Redoute, French Connection, Zara, Oasis, L.K. Bennett.

WORKING THE LOOK: SJP, Cheryl Cole, Agyness Deyn and Elizabeth Hurley.

225

5 *opulent options*

THE PERFECT AUTUMN/WINTER LOOK FOR: anyone who likes to wear special fabrics on special nights out.

GOK'S STYLE GLOSSARY: styles embellished with sequins, stones and crystals add a sprinkling of glittery glam to dark winter tones.

GET THE LOOK: if that black party dress that you pull out every Christmas is looking a little tired, why not change tack this year? Instead of going for traditional gold and silver embellishment, think about shiny black sequins on black, or navy blue on blue. Or dress up a basic black shift with a gorgeous gem-encrusted cummerbund belt and carry a sequined cocktail bag. Gold and silver brocade velvet evening jackets are also a great way to add instant glam to basic black outfits. And there should always be a place for a glistening metallic shoe in any wardrobe, as far as I'm concerned!

ESSENTIAL EXTRAS: Pile on as many of your jewels as you like – whether dangly earrings, statement necklaces, jet-bead bracelets or a gem-encrusted belt.
GOK'S STYLE TIP: black cardies covered in black sequins are a great office-to-party staple. Wear a camisole underneath and button it to just above the bust. It will instantly dress up trousers, skirts or dresses with a flash of night-time glam. You can wear it in the day, too – this is subtle shine!

SHOP THE LOOK: Monsoon, Reiss, French Connection, Mango, New Look, Primark, Topshop, Miss Selfridge, Oasis, House of Fraser.

WORKING THE LOOK: Judi Dench, Sarah Jessica Parker and Meryl Streep.

A black tux will look sensational casually thrown over your dress.

Pile on the jewels – softly shimmering baubles make for subtle shine.

227

Go for clashing colours – it's a great way to individualise your style.

WORK YOUR WARDROBE

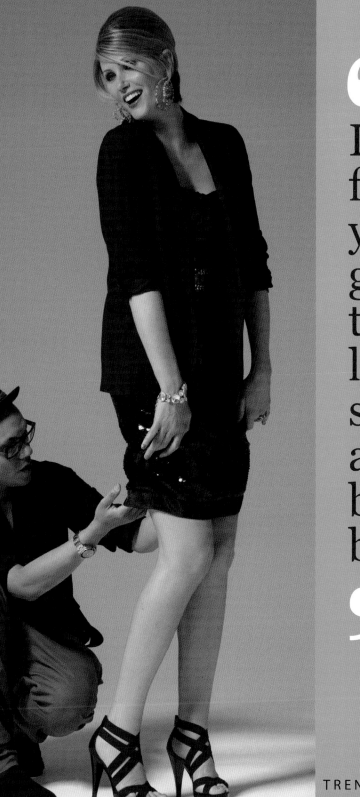

"
In these
fab looks,
you are
going
to shine
like the
stars you
are, my
beautiful
belles.
"

229

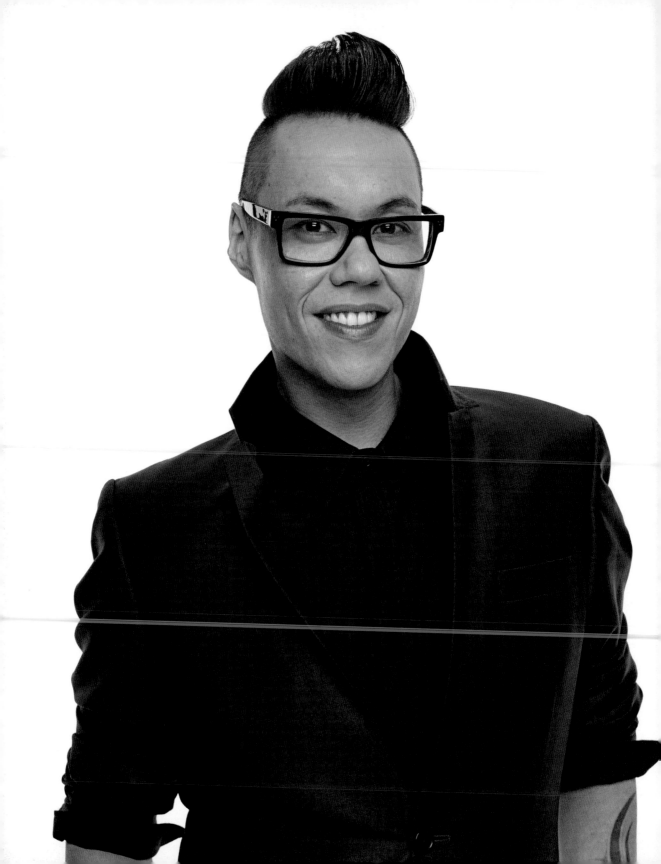

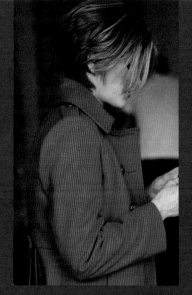

A little *word* about ...
WINTER COLOUR

NOW, MY DARLING DIVAS, JUST BECAUSE THE DARKER NIGHTS ARE ON THE WAY DOES NOT MEAN THAT YOU HAVE TO FOLLOW SUIT AND START DRESSING FOR A GOTH REVIVAL. It used to be fashion's favourite shade, but dressing in top-to-toe black can look dated now, so this winter keep thinking about adding a splash of colour to outfits. I know that black is always the easiest thing to pull on, but it can make pale skin tones look washed out. Also, all-black outfits can make any figure look shapeless, so structure outfits with accessories (gilt bracelets, necklaces and belts add instant chic to black) or jewel-tone tops and cardies (think emerald green, amethyst and sapphire). Touches of animal print look so elegant in winter: a leopard- or zebra-print cardie or skinny belt is a versatile addition to any winter wardrobe. A foxy pair of leopard-print heels is great for those office-to-party dos, and just like you, gorgeous, they'll look divine on the dance floor!

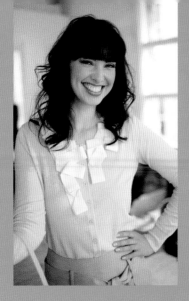

*A little **word** about ...*

DRESSING BETWEEN SEASONS

AS THE SEASONS CHANGE AND THE WEATHER BLOWS HOT AND COLD, GETTING THE BALANCE RIGHT CLOTHING-WISE IS TRICKY. If it's too warm for a winter coat, then a chunky-knit cardie-coat is a good choice. Fine knitwear, such as soft, long-sleeved delicate knits, also come in really handy at this time of year, girls, because they keep you warm but they are also easy to layer under lighter jackets. Your mac is the ideal cover-up in autumn: it's not too bulky, will keep you warm and dry, and is as stylish a windcheater as you are likely to find this side of the Arctic. It's also a good idea to work any of your big soft-knit scarves into your look now; they can be wrapped over your shoulders or draped casually round your neck.

232

A little word about ...
PREPARING YOUR WARDROBE FOR WINTER

RAINY AUTUMN SUNDAYS ARE THE IDEAL TIME TO TRANSFORM YOUR WARDROBE INTO A WINTER DRESSING-UP BOX. Start by hauling everything out and separating jackets, trousers, T-shirts, dresses and so on into orderly piles. Take a good look at all your lighter summer clothing, such as tees, shorts and sandals, and decide if you will get more wear out of them next year. If not, bin them or take them to the charity shop. Put holiday gear and summer staples, such as capri pants and good cotton shirts, into storage bags and pack them away. And bin the flip-flops, girls: they are not meant to last and will look shabby at the end of summer. But don't be so hasty when it comes to summer dresses and skirts – floral and printed ones can look really cool when worn with thick matt-black or coloured tights in winter. Also hang on to denim and leather jackets: they can be warmed up with scarves and look great with dresses and skirts in autumn. Light white and neutral-toned jackets can jar with darker autumn/winter shades, though, and are worth packing away. So too is anything that won't keep you warm – even fashion has to get practical sometimes.

233

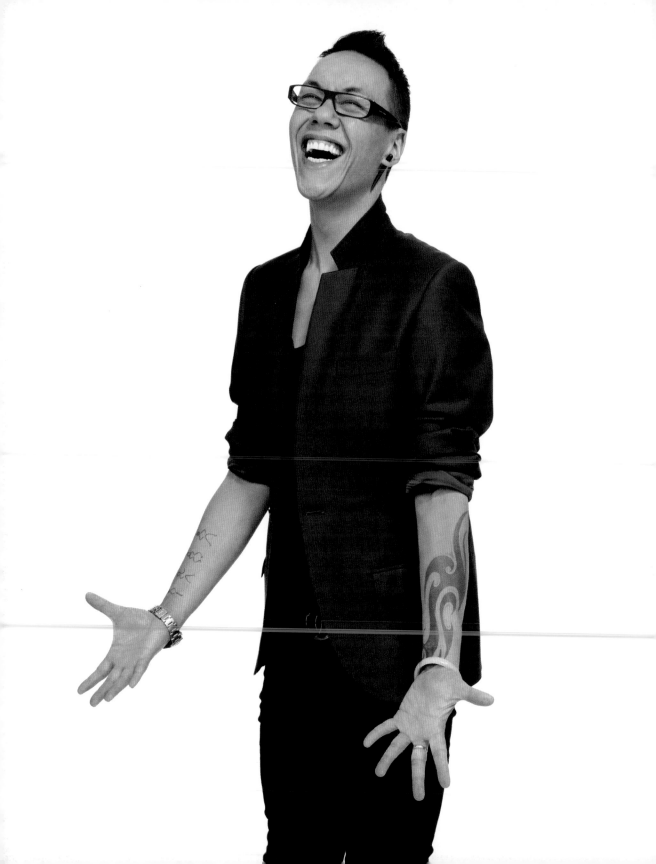

"

So, my winter angels, whether it's a day at the office, a country walk or a fabulous festive ball to get glammed up for, you're sure to have fun playing around with these winter trends. You've got your winter wardrobe stylishly wrapped up!

"

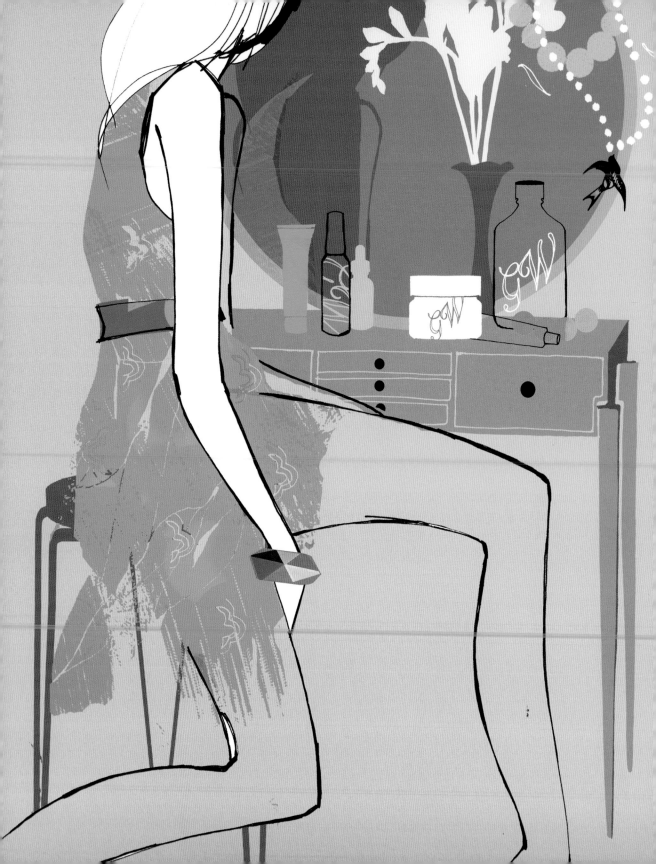

simply gorgeous

Add polish to those sassy new styles and highlight your looks with my top hair and make-up tips

beauty

MANY OF THE GIRLS I MEET ADMIT THAT, WHEN IT COMES TO RETHINKING THEIR WARDROBE, THE IDEA OF CHANGING THEIR HAIR AND MAKE-UP AT THE SAME TIME DOESN'T REALLY CROSS THEIR MIND. But, ladies, all this revitalisation is not just about getting some fresh ideas for great new looks – a style overhaul should be wholly uplifting. So, whether you like barely there make-up or want to learn how to glam up in an instant, this section is all about making more of your natural beauty.

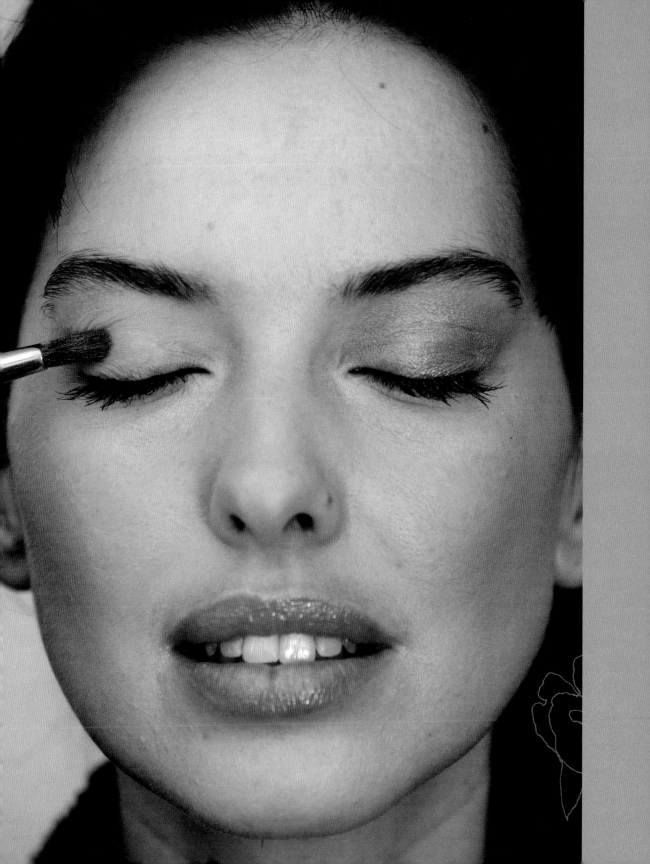

Gok's get-up-and-go beauty kit

BEING A MAKE-UP ARTIST MAY SOUND LIKE ONE OF THE MOST FABULOUS JOBS ON THE PLANET (believe me, ladies, as a former hair and make-up artist, it's not as glamorous as it seems!), but it's like any trade – you can't do the job without an up-to-date toolkit. So, ladies, just as we cleared the clutter from your wardrobe in Section One, we're going to start this chapter by spring-cleaning your beauty box, and paring it down to the basics that will work for all your beauty needs. **Here's my ESSENTIAL KIT LIST:**

1. SKINCARE

No surprises here, but regardless of skin type, you need a good everyday cleanser, eye-make-up remover and moisturiser to keep skin looking tip-top. You might also like to use a toner,

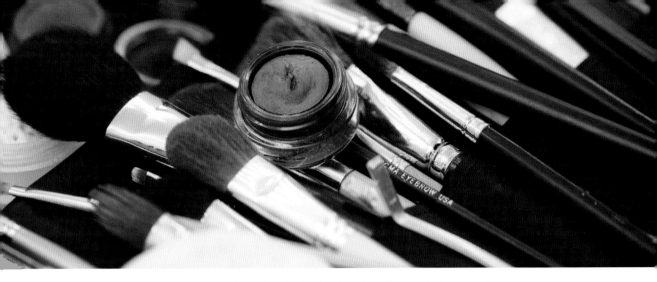

especially if your skin is oily. I don't think there's a huge difference between gentle facial washes and cleansing creams; you just need to listen to what your skin is telling you: if it feels tight, switch to something that is less drying. Also, don't feel you need to spend a fortune on expensive lotions and creams: basics such as E45 Cream and Simple Conditioning Eye-Make-Up Remover are great for all skin types. At night, really massage in that moisturiser to give skin a concentrated moisture surge.

2.MAKE-UP BRUSHES

Of all the pieces in your make-up bag, girls, brushes are the most important. In fact, I'd say that you should spend more on your brushes than you would on your make-up, as they blend make-up in well, giving it an altogether more professional look. I have to be honest here – cheaper ones will not do the trick, as they are likely just to spread liquid around the face and not blend it in. You only need to buy one or two. Expect to pay around £16 for a good eye-shadow brush, £25 for a foundation brush, £30 for a powder brush and £13 for a lip brush. If you look after them, they should last a lifetime. Try MAC Cosmetics at Maccosmetics.co.uk for some of the best.

3. MAKE-UP

• *Foundation and concealer*

Whether you like to wear make-up every day or just need the odd touch-up every now and again, a good **concealer** or **foundation** is a must for giving your complexion a balanced tone. All my girls tell me how tricky it can be to find the right one for their skin. My best tip here, sweethearts, is to consider a sheer foundation: it will give you a softer, more modern look than crème ones and you can slowly build colour over uneven areas.

• *Blusher*

Just a sweep of a pinky- or apricot-coloured **blush powder** or a **shimmery bronzer** will lift your skin. **Blush sticks** and **gels** also give a youthful glow. Apply to the apples of the cheeks and then blend outwards. Beware of darker blush shades if you're fair, as they are best used for shading areas such as the jawbone, but will enhance dark shadows elsewhere.

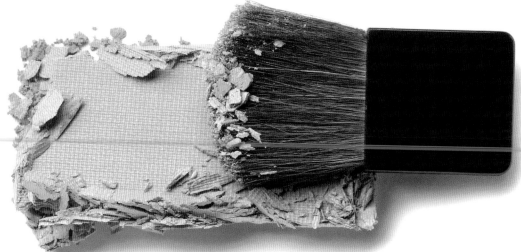

242

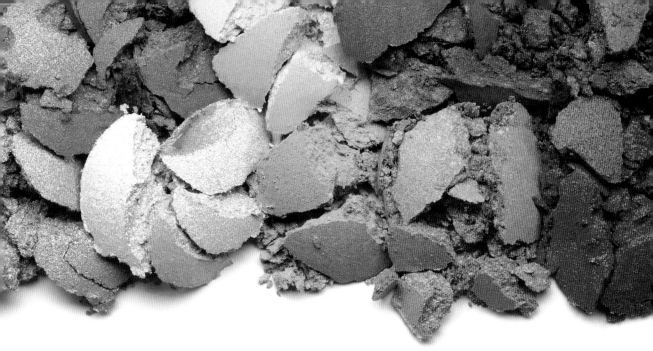

- *Eye shadow*

How many eye shadows do you have in your make-up bag right now? Too many, right, gorgeous? Well, though it may be hard for some of you beautyholics out there, my advice would be to whittle your shadows down to two. Or three – max! Even better, keep it to one palette with two or three shades in it. You can get a whole set of looks from just two shadows: simply use your blending brush and slowly build up the colour intensity – keeping it soft and light for day and stronger at night.

- *Mascara*

Designer mascaras are all very well, and that shiny packaging is a pleasure-giving addition to any make-up bag, but for a great everyday option, Maybelline Great Lash (£5 at Boots) is my first choice. It's so good. Sweep it over the outer eyelashes for a subtle look. At night, put lashings and lashings of it on and flutter the night away!

243

BEAUTY

> *Like a fabulous pair of shoes, a gorgeous lipstick will instantly update your look.*

- *Lipstick*

Like that fabulous pair of shoes, a great lipstick is the easiest way to update your look. So carry two in your handbag – a slick of do-all sheer lip tint is easy to top up throughout the day, while a super-glam bright for night will let you know that the working day is well and truly over, beautiful!

- *Vaseline*

I wouldn't be without one of these little round tins of wonderstuff and I don't think you should be, either. Use it to soften lips or to add a natural-looking gloss. Or shape eyebrows with it. (Just the teensiest amount will do for this.) You can also use it on feet and toes to help prevent blistering in summer sandals.

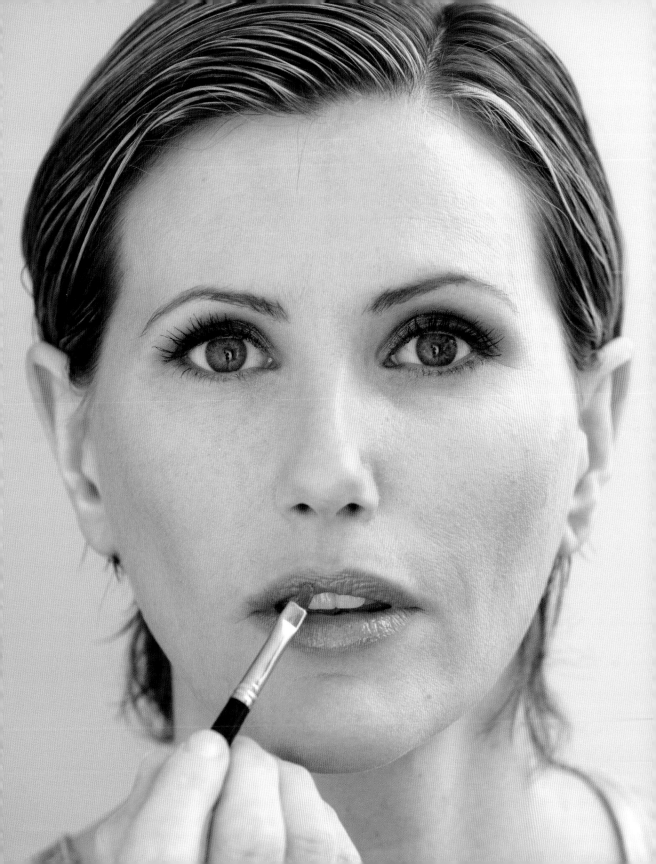

Gok's minute makeovers

Whether you've only got 10, 20, or 30 minutes to spare, I'll show you how to fit an easy make-up routine into your schedule.

10-minute girl

- **THE IDEAL ROUTINE FOR:** younger girls with low-maintenance skin, girls who don't like wearing too much make-up, mums on the run, time-strapped divas and workdays.

- **EASY EVERYDAY:** cleanse, tone and moisturise – this will instantly freshen skin. If your skin tone is uneven, brush a little concealer over redder areas or use a light-

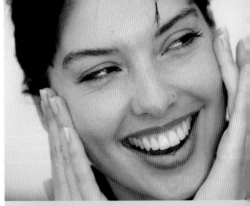

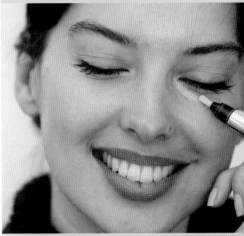

If you don't like wearing too much make-up, this is the routine for you.

coloured tinted moisturiser to even out your complexion; gently brush a light wash of neutral-tone eye shadow over the eyelid (use the same colour to shape eyebrows), draw a fine line of darker shadow with a brush or a pencil next to lashes, and lightly smudge.

Next, apply a couple of sweeps of mascara to lashes (a few more on the outer lashes will give a

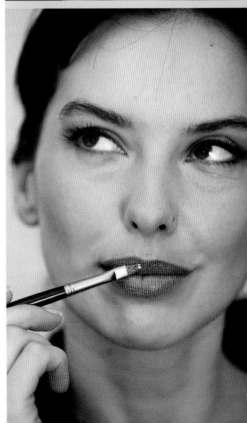

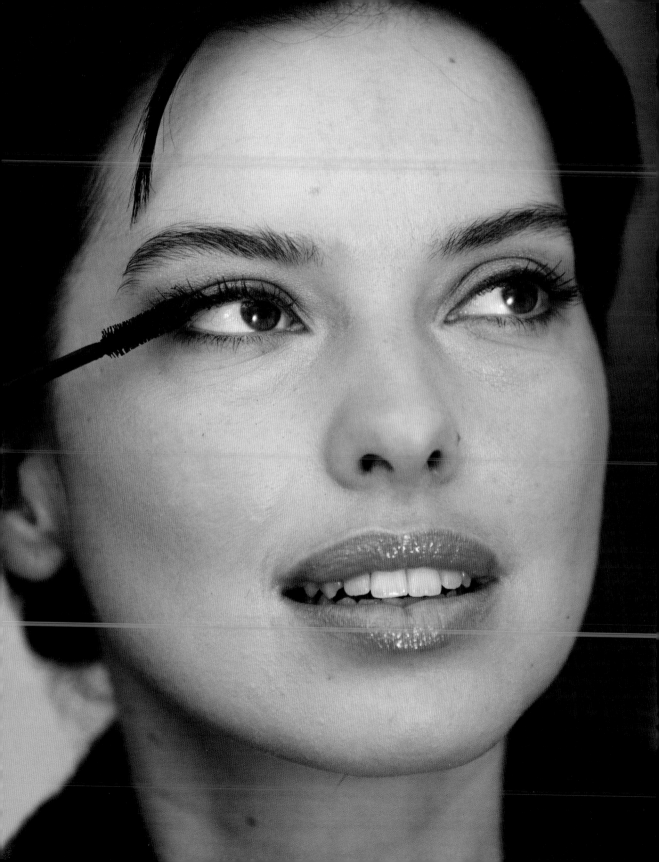

> # A day to night update is simple; add lashings of glossy mascara and a slick of lipstick in a foxier, brighter shade.

more defined effect, girls), dust a peachy blusher on the apples of the cheeks and finish off with a slick of natural gloss or Vaseline. *Et voilà!*

AFTER-DARK UPDATE: build up the eye colour and blend a darker shade in the crease of the eye or around the eyeline. Pile on the mascara and add a slick of lipstick in a foxier, brighter shade.

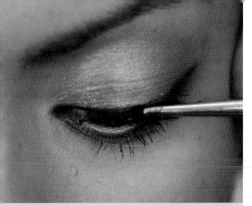

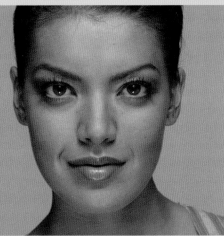

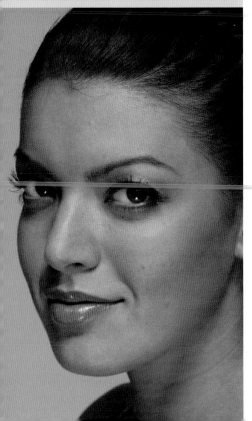

20-minute girl

- **THE IDEAL ROUTINE FOR:** thirtysomething girls who want to take a tad longer getting ready in the morning and on chilled-out weekends.

- **EASY EVERYDAY:** the idea behind this routine, ladies, is to really give your skin a nice, healthy glow by creating a good skin tone that doesn't require you whacking on a full face of foundation every day. This make-up look is all about blending – whether it's your base or your eye shadow – so that your make-up softens and flatters your features. After you've completed your skincare routine, start by just blending in the tiniest amount of concealer and then adding more gradually where you need it. Generally, you'll find the forehead, nose, chin and under-eye areas will need most attention. If you still feel that's not enough cover, then go for a tinted moisturiser – and blend, blend, blend, lady! Oh, and don't feel you have to splash out, my angel – you can always mix some foundation with your daily moisturiser and create your own instead.

Now that you've got the base sorted, you need a soft kiss of colour to lift that flawless complexion,

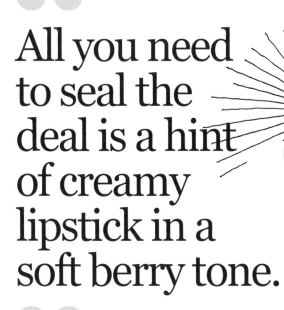

"All you need to seal the deal is a hint of creamy lipstick in a soft berry tone."

my beautiful belle, so softly brush a sweep of blusher or bronzer over your cheek-bones. Then, focusing on the eyes, apply some light-coloured eye shadow over your eyelids and blend a darker shade in along the crease. If you want more definition, you can always add more eye shadow to the outer corners of the eye – this will give you a softer effect than using eyeliner, which can look harsh in the day. You can also use your darker eye shadow to fill out your eyebrows. I think dark brown mascara is a really flattering daywear option. Now all you need to seal the deal is a hint of creamy lipstick in a soft berry tone.

> Smoky eyes are always such a hit with stars when it comes to red-carpet events, and that foxy starlet look is surprisingly easy to achieve.

• **AFTER-DARK UPDATE:** smoky eyes are always such a make-up hit at red-carpet events, and that starlet look is a surprisingly easy one to achieve. Smudge some dark eye shadow or kohl eyeliner along your upper lashes and graduate the line up towards the outer corner of the eye. If you want a more dramatic look, keep blending in eye shadow, then add lashings of mascara. Fancy a touch of sexy night-time shimmer? A sweep of bronzer over your nose, forehead and temples will do nicely. All you need now, my sultry sensation, is a sexy red-tone lip colour.

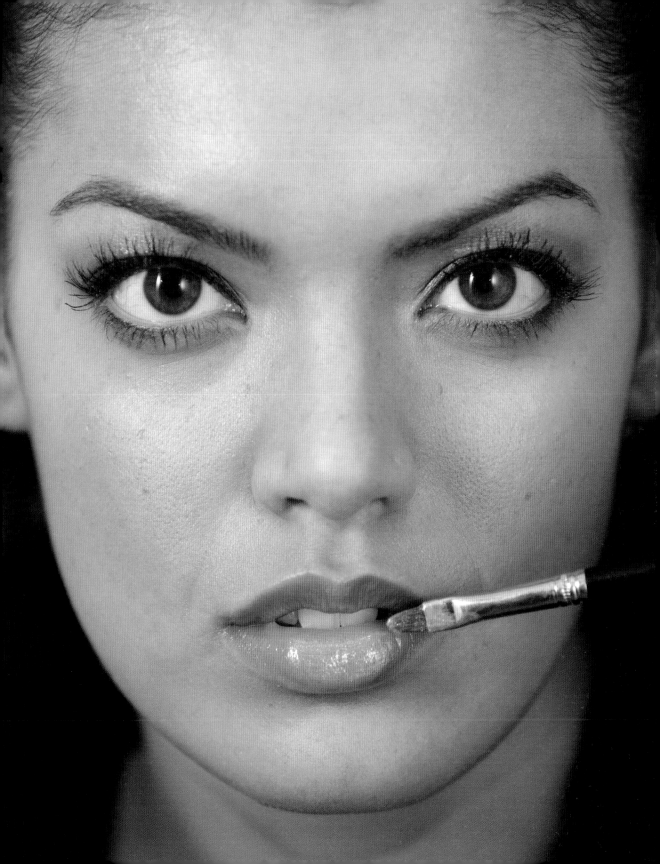

30-minute girl

- **THE IDEAL ROUTINE FOR** forty-and fiftysomething girls who like to feel gorgeously groomed; ladies who like to up the glam factor, and those days when you want to make an impression.

- **EASY EVERYDAY:** skincare is key here, ladies, so if you want your skin to feel and look as gorgeous as it can, then it's an idea to invest in richer, more specialist products. Spend as much time as you can making sure your skin feels in tip-top condition – you're worth it, my angel! Start by cleansing with a gentle product, then tone if you need to. Find a great everyday moisturiser that is not too heavy or greasy and that has inbuilt sun protection – protecting your skin from the ageing effect of the sun's rays is crucial. A light facial tanner is also a nice idea for you, as it will lift your complexion. Dot some under-eye cream below your eyes and, using an extra-light touch, gently tap the cream into the delicate skin. Drinking lots of water will flush out toxins and reduce shadows, too.

254

> **Spend as much time caring for your skin as you can. You're worth it, angel!**

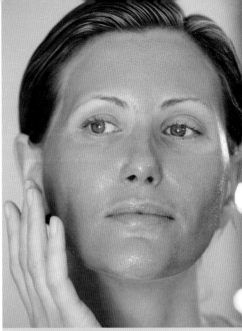

Many of my older girls are tempted to cover up using thick foundation and moisturiser, but the best way to brighten up your skin, precious, is to choose a light-reflecting foundation – these sheer formulas are designed to give your complexion a natural-looking sheen and can take years off you. (Think how much older teenagers look when they put too much make-up on – it will have exactly the same effect on you, beautiful!)

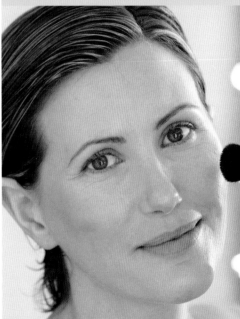

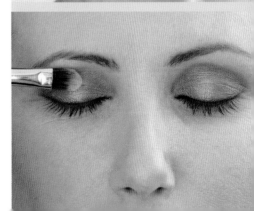

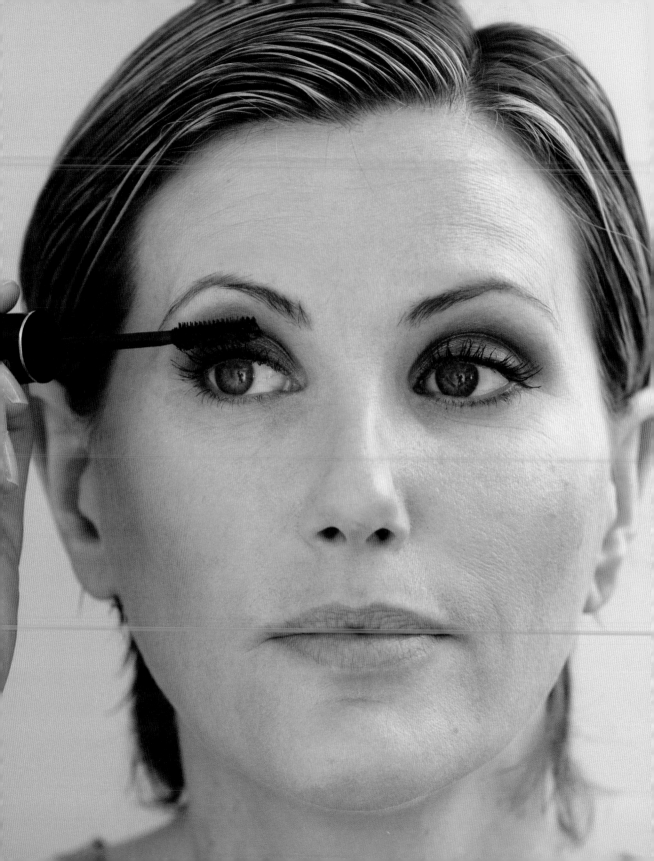

"A few of sweeps of velvety black mascara will add drama."

Use creamy products to soften your features. A few sweeps of warm-tone cream blusher, such as apricot, will instantly lift your complexion; avoid darker shades of blush unless you want to look like Frankenstein's monster! Use warm shades of cream shadow on the eyes – anything too neutral or brown can look flat. Apply liner along the upper lash line and smudge over it with one of your darker eye shadows, using an eye-shadow brush to blend both in. Use a thickening mascara to give depth to eyelashes and definitely use a lash curler if you need it. Trust me, gorgeous, it makes a huge difference.

Lastly, use a lip brush to really define the lips and sweep on some sheeny lipstick. For that full-on boardroom-belle effect, add a slick of lip gloss.

- **AFTER-DARK UPDATE:** the main trick here is to build up eye shadow so that it looks quite dark. Use more powder to build up the intensity of the look and define your eyes by blending a darker colour into the crease. A few sweeps of velvety black mascara will add drama. A soft, moisturising lip tint will subtly offset your strong eyes.

257

Gok's gorgeous make-up tips

1 IF YOU ARE GOING FOUNDATION SHOPPING, pop a hand mirror in your bag and step outside of the store so that you can get a true look at it in daylight.

2 YOU REALLY DON'T NEED TO OWN TONS OF PRODUCTS, as you can easily double them up: brown eye shadows can be used on eyebrows; lip tint can be used to colour cheeks; bronzer can be used instead of blusher. Be inventive, girls!

3 BOOK A MAKEOVER AT YOUR LOCAL DEPARTMENT STORE; it's a great way of getting a new look created by professionals for free, and it might encourage you to use products that you hadn't thought of.

4 HAVE A MAKE-UP DETOX EVERY NOW AND AGAIN – if you wear a fully made-up face every day, reduce an element every day for a week. You'll be surprised at what you can go without.

5 DON'T USE YOUR MAKE-UP AS A MASK TO HIDE BEHIND. It should be used to enhance your natural beauty, gorgeous.

6 YOUR MAKE-UP DOES NOT HAVE TO BE EXPENSIVE. Get the brushes and foundations right and you can wear what you like. Don't be bullied into buying expensive creams for daily use – keep them for pampering sessions only.

7 HAVE FUN WITH MAKE-UP; DON'T JUST ALWAYS GO FOR NATURAL LOOKS. Get bold in the evenings. And use evenings out as an excuse to get adventurous with your make-up.

259
BEAUTY

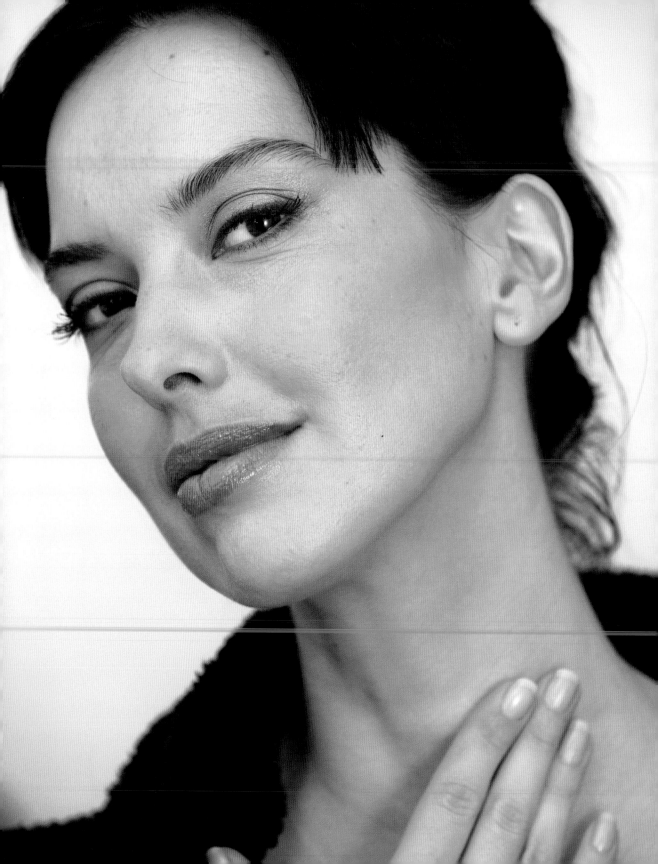

A little word about ...
BODYCARE

DON'T FORGET THAT YOUR BODY NEEDS DAILY CARE, TOO, MY BEAUTIFUL BELLES. In fact, I think this is such an important part of any revitalising routine that I was inspired to create my own Gorgeous range of body products. Nothing feels more indulgent than using a luxurious bodywash every morning, and I've packed mine with citrussy bergamot for an energising boost. Another energising tip is to switch on the cold tap just before you jump out of the shower – it will feel like torture for about two seconds, but stick with it for a few more, my ice queens, and I guarantee that it will kick-start your day like never before. Cold water gets your circulation going, helps to flush out toxins and really gets your day off to a positive start. (Those two seconds of torture are worth it, I swear!) It's also a good idea to use a softening exfoliator every couple of days; salt scrubs with essential oils will smooth skin at the same time. And moisturise your skin every day: you'll notice the difference come summer when you start baring those legs again!

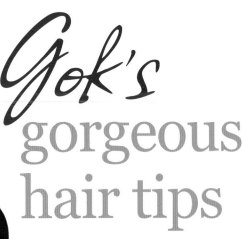

Gok's gorgeous hair tips

Well-groomed hair instantly makes you look that way, too, gorgeous, so focus on your crowning glory! Here are my top tips for luscious locks:

1 DON'T BE TEMPTED TO COVER UP YOUR FACE WITH LONG HAIR OR A HEAVY FRINGE: a good haircut will open up the face and neckline, which will have a slimming effect, too.

2 MY OLDER GIRLS MAY WANT TO CONSIDER KEEPING THEIR HAIR SHORTER: long locks can be ageing. It's that 'less is more' mantra again!

3 STRAIGHTENERS HAVE CHANGED! They are now called stylers and give a smooth, rather than a straight look. GHD are the best, as you can curl, straighten, flick, wave or crimp with them. They also come in three different sizes, so you can choose the best ones for the length or thickness of your hair.

4 INVEST IN A GOOD CONDITIONER BY A RECOGNISED BRAND, as they are unlikely to include silicones, which can build up and make hair limp.

5 IF YOU LIKE A NATURAL LOOK, REMEMBER THAT NATURAL HAIR DOESN'T HAVE TO LOOK FLAT – chestnut and golden tints will make it look shiny and healthy.

6 IF YOU ARE PALE, IT'S BEST NOT TO DYE HAIR TOO DARK OR TOO LIGHT, as either can look severe. As you get older, softer tones are the flattering option.

7 USE A THERMO-PROTECTOR SPRAY TO PREVENT HAIR FROM DRYING OUT WHEN YOU USE HEATED STYLERS – the tools will take the moisture from the protector, not your hair.

8 CHANGE YOUR HAIRDRESSER FROM TIME TO TIME: a fresh set of eyes could result in a refreshed look.

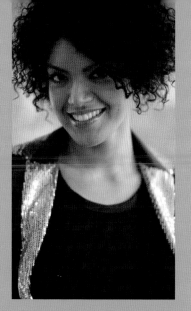

A little *word* about ...
HAIRCUTS

HAIR GROWS BY AROUND HALF AN INCH A MONTH. GET IT CUT EVERY SIX TO EIGHT WEEKS AND IT WILL ALWAYS LOOK GOOD. Take it from me, ladies, this is not just a myth invented by hairdressers to get you into the salon more: taking just a centimetre off your hair will keep your locks – and you – looking lovely and healthy. If you are growing your hair, don't be tempted to avoid your salon for months on the trot – if you don't get it trimmed regularly, by the time you go back you'll need a whole load off, as hairdryers, styling tools and the elements will have taken their terrible toll! A good hairdresser will understand that they only need to cut off a tiny amount.

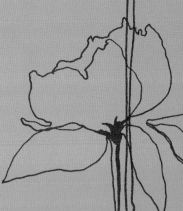

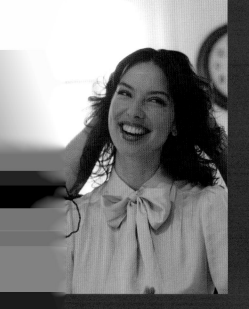

A little word about ...
HAIRSTYLES

IT CAN BE ALL TOO EASY TO CLIMB IN THAT HAIRDRESSER'S CHAIR TIME AFTER TIME AND ASK FOR THE SAME OLD STYLE. It's not so easy to get out of a hairstyle rut, though, right girls? If you're not sure how to make the change, then consider a classic cut, such as a bob. It works on every woman, from 17 to 70, and it's not all about the iconic Vidal Sassoon sixties style, either. Hairstyles are always being updated and refreshed, and the bob is a brilliant case in point. There are so many variations of it – from layered and graduated to asymmetric and inverted. Take Victoria Beckham's blonde bob reinvention a few years ago: it worked because it was level with the jawline, which made it look modern. Perhaps that's why it became one of the most requested haircuts in salons in recent times!

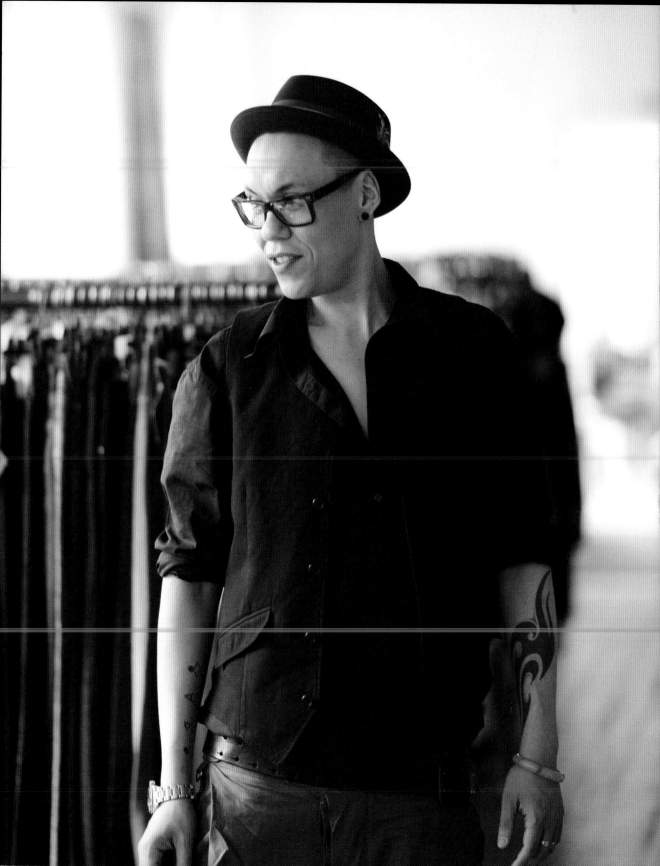

"

Now, my beautiful belles, I hope you are in your boudoir matching your outfits to your new make-up looks and that you feel more amazing than ever. All you have to do now is turn around, look in the mirror and repeat after me: 'Gorgeous, gorgeous, GORGEOUS!'

"

chapter thirteen

Gok's mini mantras

LADIES, WE ALL KNOW THAT WHEN IT COMES TO LOOKING GOOD, IT'S NOT JUST DOWN TO THE CLOTHES WE WEAR: feeling good is really important too. So, for those times when you need some inspiration, fancy a treat or just want to add instant feel-good factor to your day, here are some of my favourite FEEL-GOOD MANTRAS:

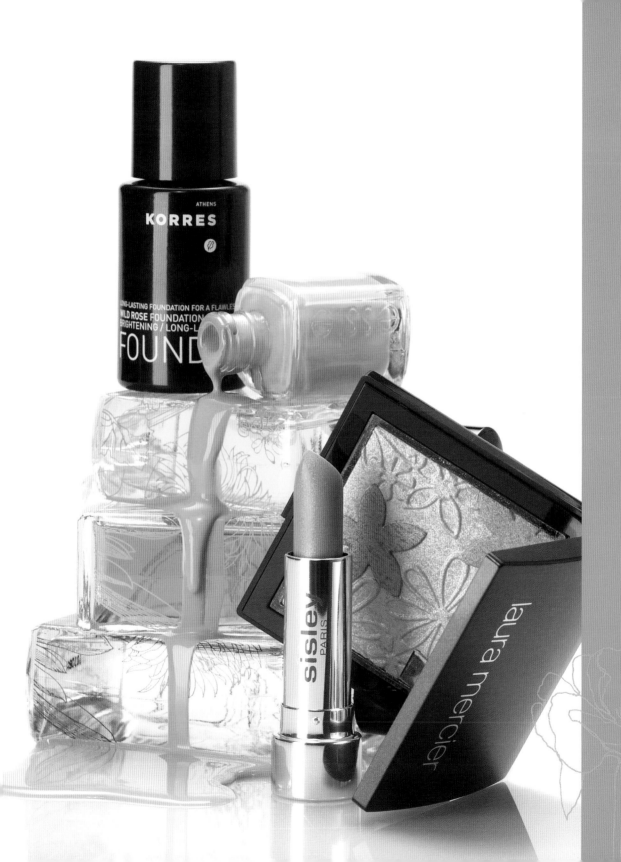

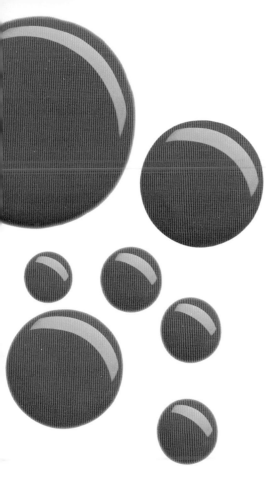

HEAVEN SCENT

ALL YOUR LOVELY MEMORIES OF HAPPY TIMES CAN BE RECAPTURED IN THE SPRITZ OF A PERFUME, so treat yourself to a scent that you love – it will always make you feel amazing.

STEP TO IT

IF YOU TEND TO WEAR SENSIBLE SHOES TO WORK EVERY DAY, wear your most fabulous heels for a change. There's nothing like a glam pair of shoes to heighten you and your day!

PERFECT POLISH

A MANICURE OR A PEDICURE IS A REAL TREAT. Book yourself in for one – or both – from time to time, and remember to choose the most opulent shade of varnish on the shelf, you decadent diva!

FUN, FUN, FUN

TRY NOT TO TAKE YOUR STYLE QUEST TOO SERIOUSLY, GORGEOUS. What you wear is an extension of how you feel – you've got to let go sometimes, and that means not worrying about getting it wrong. We all do. But, hey, so what, honey? It gives us some great photographs to look back and have a laugh at!

GOLDEN GLOW

IF YOU ARE PALE-SKINNED AND FEELING A BIT WASHED OUT, book an appointment at your local beauty salon for a spray tan, or do it at home if you have

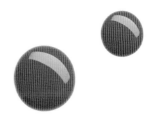

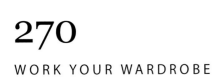

the time. There's something about a hint of summer colour that makes your mood a little sunnier, too.

● WELL FIT
DON'T MAKE YOURSELF FEEL MISERABLE BY SQUEEZING INTO CLOTHES THAT ARE TOO SMALL FOR YOU. Dress for who you are right now – honestly, beautiful, you'll look and feel so much better.

● SWEET DREAMS
NEXT TIME IT'S YOUR BIRTHDAY, ASK FOR A POT OF LUXURY FACE CREAM. Put it on every night just before you go to bed. Your skin – and you – will feel beautifully pampered, gorgeous girl.

● LIP SERVICE
DON'T SAVE WEARING A BOLDER LIP COLOUR FOR NIGHTS OUT AND SPECIAL PARTIES. A slick of bright lipstick is a great way to brighten up everyday outfits – and your mood.

● GLAMOURAMA
ORGANISE A *SEX AND THE CITY* CLOTHES-SWAP PARTY ON A SATURDAY NIGHT. Get the girls round and rustle up some cosmopolitans. It's a great way to revamp your wardrobe and clock some style tips from Carrie and the gang while you're at it!

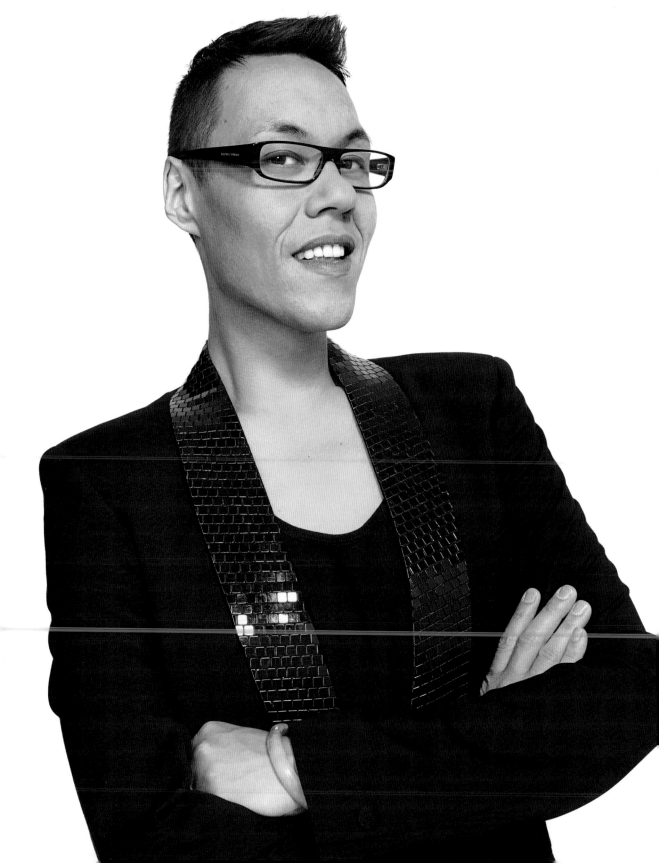

'I am fabulous and deserve to look this good.' Remember this mantra!

• COLOUR THERAPY

IF YOU FEEL IN NEED OF A COMPLETE CHANGE OF STYLE, start by choosing something in a colour that you never, ever wear. It might change the way you see your style and yourself.

• LAZY SUNDAY

TRY TO PUT ASIDE AN HOUR EVERY SUNDAY TO HAVE A MINI PAMPER SESSION: run a bath, take a stack of glossy mags into the bathroom with you and have a long, leisurely soak. For a really fabulous treat, sprinkle rose petals in the bathwater, put on a face mask and, most of all, beautiful, just relax.

• BECAUSE YOU'RE WORTH IT

EVERY MORNING, JUST BEFORE YOU LEAVE THE HOUSE, look at yourself in a full-length mirror and say, 'I am fabulous and I deserve to look this good.'

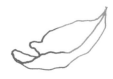

SO, MY BEAUTIFUL BABES, HOW GREAT DOES YOUR WARDROBE LOOK NOW? COOL, CLASSIC AND CHIC – JUST LIKE YOU, GORGEOUS! You should be feeling so pleased with yourselves, you fabulous fashionistas: by just whipping that wardrobe into shape, you have created a whole new set of outfits, refreshed your look and boosted your style confidence by a few notches, too. Now, whatever the occasion, you have all the components you need to put together a sensational outfit every time. Rest assured these classic styles will always look amazing, whether you are stepping out in them today, tomorrow or ten years from now.

So, my gorgeous girls, you've just proved why no one has to spend a fortune to look a million dollars – and you look right on the money, honey!

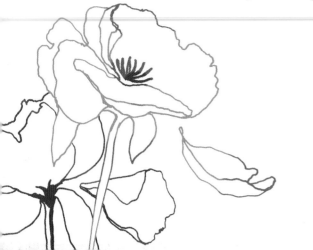

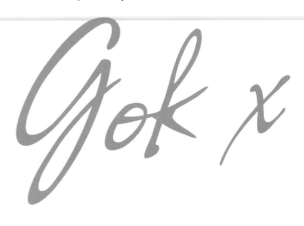

Gok x

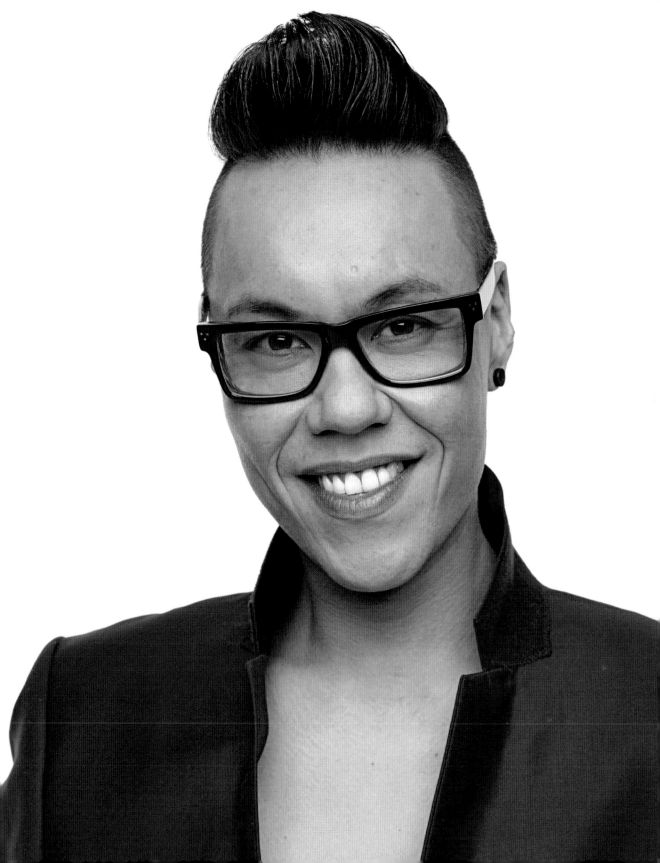

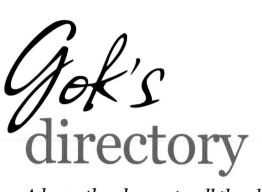

Gok's directory

A huge thank-you to all the shops who supplied us with their lovely clothes. Here's where they came from:

● section one **CHIC CLASSICS**

CHAPTER ONE: THE WHITE SHIRT (PAGES 28–9)

1. The Classic (Monica)

Earrings: Freedom at Topshop; shirt: Thomas Pink; belt: Kew; ring: The Jewellery Channel; jeans: Calvin Klein; bangles: Angie Gooderham and Lola Rose; clutch bag: Miss Selfridge; shoes: Terry de Havilland.

2. The Pussy Bow (Saffi)

Shirt: Austin Reed; brooch: vintage, Portobello Market; belt: Gap; trousers: H&M; necklaces: Heaven & Earth; bangles: Angie Gooderham; bag: Warehouse; shoes: Terry de Havilland.

3. The Classic (Carrelyn)

Scarf: Beyond Retro; shirt: Thomas Pink; belt: Stephen Collins; jeans: Debenhams; clutch bag: Russell & Bromley; shoes: New Look.

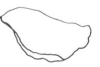

4. The Wrapover (Saffi)

Headscarf and earrings: Wallis; shirt: 'The Perfect White Shirt' at Perfekcija; jeans: Banana Republic; shoes: Strutt Couture.

5. The Pussy Bow (Monica)

Earrings: Freedom at Topshop; shirt: Jaeger; belt: Warehouse; skirt: Jaeger; bracelets: Angie Gooderham; fishnet tights: Jonathan Aston at mytights.com; shoes: ASOS.

CHAPTER TWO: JEANS (PAGES 46–7)

1. The Bootcut (Carrelyn)

Jacket: Vivienne Westwood Anglomania; blouse: Littlewoods Direct; belt: Heaven & Earth; jeans: J Brand Jeans; boots: Russell & Bromley.

2. The Skinny (Monica)

Hat: Failsworth Hats; necktie: Thomas Pink; stripy top: H&M; belt: Hobbs; jeans: Gap; shoes: Russell & Bromley.

3. The Straight (Saffi)

Blouse: By Malene Birger; jeans: Pepe; shoes: Steve Madden.

4. The Flare (Monica)

Necklace: Angie Gooderham; fringe waistcoat: Mango; vest: Gap; belt: Guess; jeans: Levi's;

bracelets: Angie Gooderham; ring: Lola Rose; shoes: Russell & Bromley.

5. The Skinny (Saffi)

Hat: Beyond Retro; necklace: Bulatti; jacket: Arrogant Cat; blouse: By Malene Birger; jeans: 7 For All Mankind; clutch bag: Russell & Bromley; shoes: Ravel.

CHAPTER THREE: TROUSERS (PAGES 66–7)

1. The Capri (Saffi)

Shirt: Uniqlo; trousers: Wallis; shoes: Limited Collection at Marks & Spencer.

2. The Wide Leg (Monica)

Hat: Beyond Retro; earrings: Freedom at Topshop; knitwear: Hoss Intropia and Brooks Brothers (worn over shoulders); gloves: Dents; trousers with belt: NW3 at Hobbs; shoes: Hobbs.

3. The Wide Leg (Carrelyn)

Earrings: Freedom at Topshop; jumper: Pringle; belt: Jigsaw; trousers: Mango; white bangle: Angie Gooderham; gold bangle: New Look; shoes: Dune.

4. The Straight (Saffi)

Jacket: Jaeger Black; silver necklace: Oasis;

black necklace: Coast; pearl necklace and vest: By Malene Birger; trousers: Jaeger Black; clutch bag: Russell & Bromley; watch: Guess; shoes: Terry de Havilland.

5. The Capri (Monica)

Necklace: Butler & Wilson; cardigan: Queene and Belle; vests: Selected Femme at House of Fraser; green bangle: Angie Gooderham; ivory bangles: Lola Rose; trousers: Dorothy Perkins; bag: Bally; shoes: Marks & Spencer.

CHAPTER FOUR: TOPS (PAGES 84–5)

1. The T-Shirt (Monica)

Sunglasses: Diesel at Safilo; earrings: Freedom at Topshop; denim jacket: Levi's; T-shirt: Dorothy Perkins; skinny jeans: Warehouse; shoes: Faith.

2. The Belted Cardigan (Carrelyn)

Hat: Failsworth Hats; pearls: Angie Gooderham; cardigan: Banana Republic; vest: Miss Selfridge; belt: Jigsaw; trousers: Mango; pumps: Gap.

3. The Vest (Saffi)

Earrings: Erickson Beamon; vest: Ghost; blade bracelet: Angie Gooderham; disco-ball bracelet: Erickson Beamon; studded bracelet,

belt and sequinned pencil skirt: By Malene Birger; shoes: Reiss.

4. The Cardigan (Monica)

Earrings: Erickson Beamon; cardigan: Jigsaw; skirt: Wallis; gloves: Dents; bag: Russell & Bromley; shoes: Oasis.

5. The Waistcoat (Saffi)

Denim waistcoat: Wrangler; check shirt: New Look; jeans: PRPS; shoes: Keds.

CHAPTER FIVE: DRESSES & SKIRTS (PAGES 106–7)

1. The Mini Shift Dress (Monica)

Hat: Failsworth Hats; red shift dress: Jesiré; belt: Hobbs; gloves: Guess Jeans; bag: Jaeger; tights: Trasparenze at mytights.com; boots: Dune.

2. The Wrap Dress (Carrelyn)

Necktie: Zara; dress: Diane von Furstenberg at Matches; belt: Oasis; bag: Russell & Bromley; boots: Clarks.

3. The Pencil Skirt (Saffi)

Earrings: Freedom at Topshop; denim jacket: Levi's; T-shirt: Junk Food; black pencil skirt: Diva Corsets; clutch bag: Miss Selfridge; bangles: Freedom at Topshop; tights: Jonathan Aston at mytights.com; boots: Peacocks.

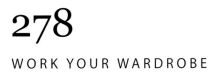

4. The Wide Skirt (Monica)

Hairband: Topshop; jacket: Paul Costelloe Collection at House of Fraser; necklace: Erickson Beamon; vest: Miss Selfridge; belt: Bally; skirt: Gia London; shoes: Steve Madden.

5. The Shift Dress (Saffi)

Hat: Full Circle; scarf: Accessorize; dress: Hobbs; belt: Warehouse; gloves: Dents; tights: Jonathan Aston at mytights.com; boots: Dune.

CHAPTER SIX: JACKETS & COATS (PAGES 128–9)

1. The Mac (Monica)

Scarf: Accessorize; mac: Lipsy; shirt: Brooks Brothers; belt: Heaven & Earth; jeans: Levi's; loafers: Kate Kuba.

2. The Blazer (Saffi)

Scarf: Accessorize; blazer: Heaven & Earth; stripy cardigan: Hobbs; shorts: Banana Republic; belt: Marks & Spencer; bag: Jasper Conran for Debenhams; shoes: George at Asda.

3. The Military Coat (Monica)

Hat: Failsworth Hats; coat: Vivienne Westwood Anglomania; black belt: Warehouse; fabric belt: Beyond Retro; gloves: Oasis; tights: Trasparenze at mytights.com; patent ankle boots: Russell & Bromley.

4. The Blazer (Carrelyn)

Sunglasses: Hugo Boss at Safilo; blazer: Austin Reed; T-shirt: Junk Food; jeans: A\Wear; bag: Warehouse; shoes: Faith.

5. The Boyfriend Blazer (Saffi)

Earrings: Erickson Beamon; blazer: Gerard Darel; dress: Oasis; bracelet: Butler & Wilson; shoes: ASOS.

●section two
ELEGANT EXTRAS

CHAPTER SEVEN: SHOES & BOOTS

Ballet Pumps (page 142)

Fluorescent yellow: Pretty Ballerinas; pink: Gap; red with bow: Marks & Spencer; turquoise with bow: Pretty Ballerinas.

Riding Boots (page 149)

Hat: Failsworth Hats; red jacket: A\Wear; black dress: Almost Famous Ltd; tights: Trasparenze at mytights.com; riding boots: De Niro Boots.

Ankle Boot (page 150)

Green strappy ankle boot: Kate Kuba.

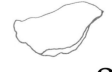

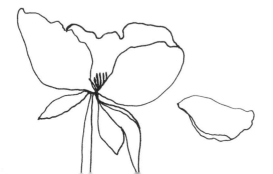

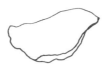

brown satchel: Pepe Jeans; brown pumps: Jones Bootmaker.

3. Brilliant Black and White (page 203)

Dress: Hobbs; brooch: Butler & Wilson; sunglasses: H&M; bag: Heaven & Earth; shoes: Debenhams.

4. Second Skin (page 204)

Headband: NW3 at Hobbs; earrings: Butler & Wilson; necklace: Freedom at Topshop; belt: By Malene Birger (worn across top); nude jumpsuit: gorgeouscouture.com; link bracelet: Butler & Wilson; disco bangle: Erickson Beamon; silver bangle: Angie Gooderham; shoes: Reiss.

5. Fabulous Florals (page 207)

Sunglasses: Dior Eyewear; earrings: New Look; dress: Hoss intropia; ring: Lola Rose; bag: Russell & Bromley; shoes: Faith.

CHAPTER ELEVEN: TRENDS AUTUMN/WINTER

1. Military Mode (page 219)

Snood: Oasis; jacket: H&M; gloves: Oasis; trousers: Gap; bag: Jaeger; shoes: Oasis.

2. Glamorous Gowns (Carrelyn, page 220)

Earrings: Butler & Wilson; dress:

gorgeouscouture.com; brooch: Erickson Beamon; clutch bag: Dents; shoes: New Look.

3. Foxy Fringing (Carrelyn, page 223)

Dress: By Malene Birger; stockings: Aristoc at mytights.com; shoes: Hobbs.

4. Bolts of Colour (Monica, page 224)

Hat: Kangol; blouse: Jaeger; belt: Stephen Collins; skirt: Jaeger; ring: Lola Rose; clutch bag: Miss Selfridge; tights: Jonathan Aston at mytights.com; shoes: Terry de Havilland.

5. Opulent Options (page 227)

Earrings: Erickson Beamon; jacket: Gerard Darel; dress: NW3 at Hobbs; belt: By Malene Birger; shoes: Office; jewelled clutch bag: Dents.

• section four
SIMPLY GORGEOUS

CHAPTER TWELVE: BEAUTY

Gok's Mini Mantras Shot (page 269)

Wild Rose foundation: Korres; pink nail polish: Essie; Coeur de Fleur Eau de Toilette: Miller Harris; Noix de Tubereuse Eau de Parfum: Miller Harris; Usiku Organic Eau de Toilette: Jo Wood Organics; Phyto-Lip Shine: Sisley; blusher compact: Laura Mercier

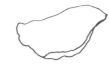

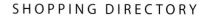

where to buy

Styles referred to in this book:

a

A\Wear: 00 35 3724956, www.awear.com

Accessorize: 0844 811 0069, www.monsoon.co.uk

All Saints: 0870 458 3736, www.allsaints.com

Almost Famous Ltd: 020 7637 2622, www.aflondon.com

Angie Gooderham: 020 7488 0935, www.angie-gooderham.co.uk

A.P.C. at Net-a-porter 08456 75 13 21, www.net-a-porter.com

Arrogant Cat: 020 7323 0886, www.arrogantcat.com

ASOS: www.asos.com

Austin Reed: 01845 573 135, www.austinreed.co.uk

b

Baccarat: available at Harrods 0845 605 1234, www.harrods.com

Bally: 020 7408 9877, www.bally.com

Banana Republic: 08457 697 072, www.bananarepublic.eu

Betty Jackson Black: available at Debenhams, 08445 616 161, www.debenhams.com

Beyond Retro: 020 7613 3636, www.beyondretro.com

Blowfish: available at Rubber Sole, www.rubbersole.co.uk

Brogini: 01706 340500, www.brogini.com

Brooks Brothers: 020 7238 0030, www.brooksbrothers.com

Bulatti: 01245 360949, www.bulatti.co.uk

Butler & Wilson: 020 7409 2955, www.butlerandwilson.co.uk

By Malene Birger: available at Net-a-Porter, 08456 75 13 21, www.net-a-porter.com

c

Calvin Klein Jeans: 020 7580 1327, www.calvinkleinjeans.com

Carvela: available at Kurt Geiger, 0845 257 2571, www.kurtgeiger.com

Charles Tyrwhitt: 0845 337 3 337, www.ctshirts.co.uk

Chloé, at My Wardrobe: 0845 260 3880; www.my-wardrobe.com

Clarks: 0844 4777744, www.clarks.co.uk

Coast: 0845 899 1119, www.coast-stores.co.uk

Converse, available at Office: 0845 058 0777, www.office.co.uk

d

Debenhams: 08445 616 161,
www.debenhams.com
De Niro Boots: available at Brogini, 01706
340500, www.brogini.com
Dents: 01985 212 291, www.dents.co.uk
Diane von Furstenberg: available at Matches,
0870 067 8838, www.matchesfashion.com
Diesel: 020 7520 7799, www.diesel.com
Diva Corsets: 01491 628 844, www.divacorsets.com
Dorothy Perkins: 0844 984 0264,
www.dorothyperkins.com
Dune: 020 7636 8307, www.dune.co.uk

e

Erickson Beamon: 0207 259 0202,
www.ericksonbeamon.com
Essie: available at Nails by Mail,
0844 800 9396, www.nailsbymail.co.uk

f

Failsworth Hats: 0161 681 3131,
www.failsworth-hats.co.uk
Faith: 0800 289 297, www.faith.co.uk
Freedom: available at Topshop 0870 606 9666,
www.topshop.com
French Connection: 0844 557 3285,
www.frenchconnection.com
Fullcircle: 020 8753 0112,
www.fullcircleuk.com

g

Gap: 0800 427 789, www.gap.com
George at Asda: 0500 100055,
www.asda.com/george

Gerard Darel: 0207 586 9027,
www.gerarddarel.com
Gia: 020 8245 5226, www.gia-london.com
Ghost: 0800 008 7772, www.ghost.co.uk
Gorgeouscouture.com: 0845 331 3320,
www.gorgeouscouture.com
Guess: 020 7240 2086, www.guess.com
Guess Watches: available at British Watch
Company, 02476 555 526,
www.britishwatchcompany.com

h

Heaven & Earth: 0207 468 6090,
www.heavenandearthclothing.com
Hobbs: 020 7586 5550, www.hobbs.co.uk
Hoss intropia: available at Yoox,
0800 046 3688, www.yoox.com
House of Fraser: 0845 602 1073,
www.houseoffraser.co.uk
H&M: 020 7323 2211, www.hm.com

i

Issa: available at Matches 0870 067 8838,
www.matchesfashion.com

j

J Brand jeans: available at My Wardrobe,
0845 260 3880, www.my-wardrobe.com
Jaeger: 0845 051 0063, www.jaeger.co.uk
Jas M.B.: 020 7494 2288, www.jas-mb.com
Jesire: 020 7420 4459, www.jesire.net
Jigsaw: 020 7437 5750,
www.jigsaw-online.com
Jones Bootmaker: 0800 163 519,
www.jonesbootmaker.com

Jo Wood Organics: 0845 607 6614, www.jowoodorganics.com
Juicy Couture: available at Net-a-porter: 08456 75 13 21, www.net-a-porter.com
Junk Food: available at Truffle Shuffle, 0117 982 8884, www.truffleshuffle.co.uk

k

Kangol: 01946 818350, www.kangolstore.com
Karen Millen: 0845 899 4449, www.karenmillen.com
Kate Kuba: 020 7715 5303, www.katekuba.co.uk
Keds: available at Rubber Sole: www.rubbersole.co.uk
Kew: 020 8487 2000, www.kew-online.com
Korres: 020 7581 6455, www.korres.com
Kurt Geiger: 0845 257 2571, www.kurtgeiger.com

l

Lacoste: 020 7491 8968, www.lacoste.com
Laura Mercier: available at Selfridges, 0800 123 400, www.selfridges.com
Lee jeans: 020 7193 3996, www.lee-store.com
Levi's: 01604 599735, www.levistrauss.com
Lipsy: 0844 844 0088, www.lipsy.co.uk
Littlewoods: 0844 822 8000, www.littlewoods.com
L. K. Bennett: 0844 581 5881, www.lkbennett.com
Lola Rose: 020 7372 0777, www.lolarose.co.uk

m

Mango: 0845 082 2448, www.mangoshop.com
Marc by Marc Jacobs, at Matches: 0870 067 8838, www.matchesfashion.com
Marks & Spencer: 0845 302 1234, www.marksandspencer.com
Miller Harris: 0844 561 0992, www.millerharris.com
Miss Selfridge: 0844 984 0263, www.missselfridge.com
Miss Sixty: www.misssixty.com
Monsoon: 0844 811 0068, www.monsoon.co.uk
My Tights: 020 7819 0530, www.mytights.com
My Wardrobe: 0845 260 3880, www.my-wardrobe.com

n

Net-a-porter: 08456 75 1321, www.net-a-porter.com
New Look: 0500 454094, www.newlook.co.uk
Next: 0870 243 5435, www.next.co.uk

o

Oasis: 0845 899 0009, www.oasis-stores.co.uk
Office: 0845 058 0777, www.office.co.uk

p

Patrick Cox: 020 7730 8886; www.patrickcox.com
Paul Costelloe: available at House of Fraser, 0845 602 1073, www.houseoffraser.co.uk
Peacocks: 029 2027 0222, www.peacocks.co.uk
Pepe Jeans: 020 7313 3800, www.pepejeans.com
Perfekcija: 020 8440 9977, www.perfekcija.co.uk
Pretty Ballerinas: 020 7493 3957,

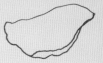

www.prettyballerinas.com
Pringle: 0800 360200,
www.pringlescotland.com

q

Queene and Belle: 01750 23419,
www.queeneandbelle.com

r

R. Soles: 0207 351 5520, www.rsoles.com
Ravel shoes: available at Freemans,
0844 556 4444, www.freemans.com
Reiss: 020 7473 9630, www.reiss.co.uk
River Island: 0844 826 9835,
www.riverisland.com
Russell & Bromley: 020 8460 1122,
www.russellandbromley.co.uk

s

Safilo: 01423 520303, www.safilo.com
Savile Row Co: 028 7946 5000,
www.savilerowco.com
Sergio Rossi: available at Net-a-Porter,
08456 75 13 21, www.net-a-porter.com
Shellys: available at Asos: www.asos.com
Sisley: 020 7591 6380,
www.sisley-cosmetics.co.uk
Stephen Collins: 020 8658 3634,
www.stephencollins.co.uk
Steve Madden: 020 7428 7428,
www.stevemadden.com
Strutt Couture: 020 7127 0007,
www.struttcouture.com
Superga: available at Rubber Sole,
www.rubbersole.co.uk

t

Terry de Havilland: 01252 730618,
www.terrydehavilland.com
The Jewellery Channel: 0844 375 4444,
www.thejewellerychannel.tv
Thomas Pink: 020 7498 3882,
www.thomaspink.com
T. M. Lewin: 0845 389 1898,
www.tmlewin.co.uk
Topman: 0844 984 0265, www.topman.com
Topshop: 0845 121 4519, www.topshop.com

u

Uniqlo: www.uniqlo.co.uk
Urban Outfitters: 0845 330 1288,
www.urbanoutfitters.co.uk

v

Vivienne Westwood Anglomania:
available at My Wardrobe, 0845 260 3880,
www.mywardrobe.com

w

Wallis: 0800 121 4520, www.wallis-fashion.com
Warehouse: 0870 1228813,
www.warehouse.co.uk
Whistles: 0870 770 4301, www.whistles.co.uk
Wrangler: available at www.asos.com
(020 7734 9223; www.wrangler.com)

z

Zara: 020 7851 4300, www.zara.com

7 For All Mankind: available at
I love Jeans, 020 8446 4299,
www.ilovejeans.com

* Please note that some shops may carry a selection of styles only and that it cannot
be guaranteed that specific items featured will be in stock at time of publication.

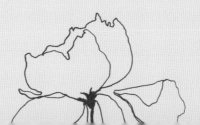

Thank You...

I would like to thank, with deepest love, my entire family for your love and guidance and never-tiring support. Without all of you I would not be able to survive. I love you all so much that sometimes it hurts, you truly are my everything.

A special thank you to my adorable nieces Maya Lily and Lola Rose, who never cease to fill my world with happiness and laughter.

Thank you to all my fabulous dear friends for allowing me to once again take leave of our special time together in order for me to work and develop. I love each of you from the bottom of my bottom!

A special squeeze to my goddaughter Yasmine, aka Joan Collins.

A huge thank you to Carol, you've become a friend, mentor and an honest place in my heart.

Thank you to all the girls and guys at HarperCollins for working so hard.

Caragh, so stylish and clever and a new girl in my life who I know I can count on whenever I need to fashion purge!

Kirsty, you are such an inspiration and a dear friend – can we get drunk now?

Nikki, headstrong and creative – my kind of girl!

Anna, such a clever girl and always the diplomat!

Alicja and Cher, the dynamic duo with such great vision.

Perou, glasses and hats are the new black!

Chris, the one to watch – behind-the-scenes glamour!

Charlie and Jamie, make-up and hair wouldn't be the same without you.

Sue Murphy, life has been unpredictable but if any girl can find reason, then it's you.

A big thank you to Theshoreditch.com who looked after us all so fabulously on our shoot week.

And finally, a huge, massive, gigantic banger-boosting snog to all my loyal Gokettes who have supported me. I will always be your Auntie Gok.

Gok x

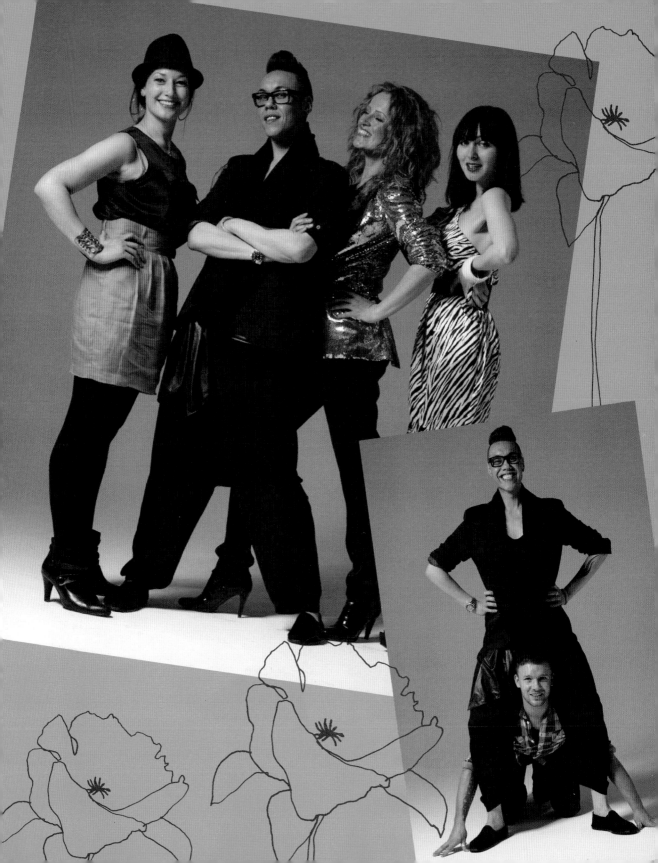

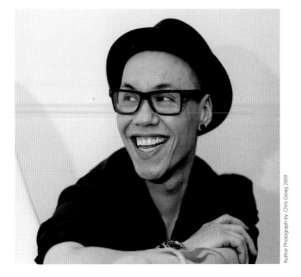

Style supremo **Gok Wan** is every woman's best friend.
He has worked in the industry for over a decade, dressing
countless celebrities and fashion pages. His TV makeover series
How to Look Good Naked transformed him into a star, not least
because he genuinely cares about the women whose style and lives
he changes. He also presents Channel 4's weekly celebration
of fashion, *Gok's Fashion Fix*. His previous two books,
How to Look Good Naked and *How to Dress*,
were instant bestsellers.

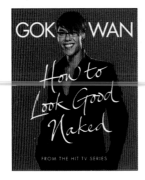
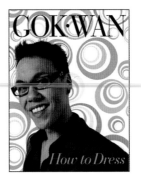